Longevity

Future of Enhanced Lifespans and Vitality

By Viktor Simunovic MD

Longevity

Copyright 2023 © (Viktor Simunovic), Longevity

Disclaimer

The information presented in this book, "Longevity: Future of Enhanced Lifespans and Vitality," is intended for educational and informational purposes only. While every effort has been made to ensure the accuracy and reliability of the content, the author and publisher do not make any representations or warranties regarding the completeness, suitability, or applicability of the information contained herein. Readers are advised to consult with qualified healthcare professionals or medical practitioners before implementing any lifestyle changes, dietary modifications, or medication regimens discussed in this book. Individual health conditions and medical needs may vary, and what works well for one person may not be suitable for another. The discussions on longevity medications, including Rapamycin, Metformin, and Acarbose, are based on current scientific research and understanding. However, the field of longevity science is constantly evolving, and new discoveries may impact the perspectives and recommendations provided in this book.

The author's opinions expressed in this book are solely their own and do not necessarily reflect the views of the publisher or other entities mentioned herein. Readers are encouraged to critically evaluate the information presented and to conduct their own research or seek professional medical advice when making decisions related to their health and well-being. The author and publisher disclaim any liability, loss, or risk incurred as a direct or indirect consequence of the use or application of any information presented in this book. By reading this book, readers agree to hold harmless the author, publisher, and any affiliated parties from any claims, damages, or injuries arising from the interpretation or implementation of the content herein. All rights reserved. No part of this publication may be reproduced, distributed, or transmitted in any form or by any means, including photocopying, recording, or other electronic or mechanical methods, without the prior written permission of the publisher, except in the case of brief quotations embodied in critical reviews and certain other noncommercial uses permitted by copyright law.

Thank you for your understanding and cooperation.

Dedication

To the seekers of wisdom and champions of vitality,

This book is dedicated to all those who dare to dream of a future where aging is not synonymous with decline, but rather an opportunity for growth, resilience, and boundless possibility.

To the pioneers of longevity science, whose unwavering commitment to discovery fuels the quest for a world where every individual can live a life of health, vitality, and purpose.

To the caregivers and healers, whose compassion and dedication illuminate the path towards holistic well-being, reminding us that the journey to longevity is not a solitary endeavor but a collective pursuit rooted in empathy and human connection.

To the visionaries and innovators, whose bold ideas and tireless efforts pave the way for transformative breakthroughs, shaping a future where the boundaries of possibility are continually redrawn.

May this book serve as a beacon of inspiration and knowledge, igniting the flames of curiosity and empowerment in all who turn its pages. May it spark conversations, challenge assumptions, and ignite a movement towards a world where aging is celebrated as a journey of growth and fulfillment.

With deepest gratitude and heartfelt appreciation,

Viktor Simunovic

About the Author

I am **Viktor**, a Doctor of Medicine (M.D.) and healthcare technology entrepreneur with a passion for innovation and improving patient care. With over a decade of experience in the field, I have dedicated my career to leveraging the latest tools and technologies to streamline operations and enhance healthcare delivery worldwide.

As the Co-Founder of EUDoctor, my mission is to address the challenges and inefficiencies prevalent in the healthcare industry. EUDoctor is not just a technical solution; it's a vision to make high-quality, multilingual healthcare and medical consultations accessible to patients irrespective of their backgrounds. Through our platform, we offer online consultations, telehealth services, telemedicine prescriptions, and sick leave notes, simplifying communication with doctors across the EU.

In addition to my role at EUDoctor, I am also a practicing General Practitioner and the proud owner of GP Clinic Viktor Simunović. At my clinic, I provide a range of primary care and healthcare services, drawing upon my expertise in Health Sciences and Dermatology to offer personalized medical care to my patients. Through GP Clinic Viktor Simunović, I extend telehealth services and pharmaceutical strategic healthcare consulting, collaborating with major European pharmacies to optimize medical solutions.

Furthermore, I am the Founder of Brave Bear, a software development company specializing in innovative solutions for the healthcare industry. Through Brave Bear, we have developed cutting-edge applications supporting telemedicine and primary care services, driving advancements in patient care and medical efficiency.

My core competencies encompass primary care, healthcare technology innovation, and the delivery of multilingual healthcare services in English, Croatian, and Italian. I am deeply committed to advancing healthcare accessibility and quality, and I am always eager to collaborate with like-minded individuals to explore new opportunities and projects.

If you're interested in learning more about my ventures or exploring collaboration opportunities, please feel free to reach out to me. I am enthusiastic about connecting with individuals who share my passion for transformative healthcare solutions and discovering exciting possibilities together.

Viktor Simunovic

Table of Contents

LONGEVITY

Viktor Simunovic

CHAPTER 1
INTRODUCTION

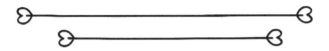

1.1. Overview of the Book

In a contemporary landscape where aging populations and the pursuit of extended vitality command both scientific inquiry and public fascination, "Longevity: Future of Enhanced Lifespans and Vitality" appears against the backdrop of dynamics between aging, health practices and state-of-the-art biomedical interventions. Informed by a coterie of luminary champions firmly grounded in the epicenter of longevity, this treatise charts an audience-centered global march toward a radical examination of what operates under the hood orchestrating aging and enabling breakthrough strategies proffering extraordinary freedom from mortal limitation.

At its core, "Longevity" is a two-edged narrative that fuses the values of healthy living with an emerging industry and wants to change lives, lengthening lives by transforming them through longevity-enhancing drugs. Divorced into two clearly demarcated entities, the book diligently unwinds the dense weft of influences formulating aging alongside hurdling into the progressive possibilities of some pharmacologic interventions.

The introductory chapter is a starting point in that it guides travelers on their journey for extended life. From its first part delve into the underlying core principles of healthy lifestyle practices it highlights the key roles that nutrition, physical activity and stress reduction with sleep play in creating whole health and wellbeing. By way of a synthesized blend in empirical evidence and pragmatic advocation, readers are encouraged to integrate these lifestyle principles into their everyday lives, thus consolidating the trajectory of their health and creating favorable conditions for long-term viability.

Biological substrates that are concealed at the center of this discourse on healthy ageing is intricate and involved. And fascination is hard to miss when you venture into the molecular complexities of cells' metabolism, or on a systemic bounce between chronic inflammation – all clearly illuminated as "Longevity" navigates the intricate abysses of aging biology. The novel helps readers understand the physiological functions of lifestyle determinants that control the aging chain, hence providing a fundamental understanding of bodily property from the foundation of which they can make rational decisions relating to their lifelong health goals.

Additionally, 'Longevity' goes beyond just elucidation and invites readers to the forefront of biomedical innovation with its discussion of pharmacological interventions set to revise the aging paradigm. Meanwhile, setting sail on an intriguing voyage through the landscape of molecular medicine, there is the disclosure of a pantheon of pharmacotherapeutic modalities such as senolytics which eliminate senescent cells and metformin's multi-faceted metabolic powers that show potential in minimizing degenerative disability and promoting optimal longevity. Nonetheless, in the midst of a feverish celebration for pharmacological miracles, "Longevity" endures its goal to continued wellness by sustaining the importance of an integration between lifestyle adherence and medication. With an understanding of the complex interrelationship between environmental triggers and pharmacodynamic reactions, this book promotes a judicious combination of lifestyle adjustments along with drug-based adjuncts adapted to personalized health pathways.

These medications marked a revolution in the field of redefining the touch points of aging as these drugs address critical pathways and processes within the body. However, rapamycin, initially planned as an organ rejection inhibitor, has gained importance owing to its capacity in enhancing life span. Its mode of operation centers around the mTOR regulative axis-a key driver of metabolism and growth. By repression mTOR, the anti-aging agent called Rapamycin interferes with central cellular processes thus enabling an attempt to block aging at its core. By deep analysis, the readers get knowledge of details at the molecular level on the rapamycin's longevity regulating mechanisms.

As another interesting option, metformin as a veteran in type 2 diabetes management may gain the capability to prolong life. Apart from being a common abridgement for glycemic control, the evolution of Metformin has shown diverse effects and functions in cellular metabolism including inflammation. The investigation of Metformin's molecular interactions as well as its therapeutic utility allows readers to acquire a multi-layered picture of the properties that make it stand out as a possible longevity molecule.

Despite the fact that acarbose is less known, it offers a remarkable and relatively unusual approach to glucagon response regulation for longevity by modulating carbohydrate metabolism and gut microbiota. Modulating the gut flora is one such mechanism through which Acarbose influences metabolic health; hence, a key component of fitness for aging and longevity. It treats corresponding metabolic processes as mechanisms not related to each other but in timber which can be considered peculiar by virtue of the fact that one process is translated into the decrease of another and vice versa.

The term "Longevity" is a masterpiece with proper balancing of scientific languages of accurate and archetypal prose for readers from all walks of life to get immersed in the intricacies of science that govern longevity. In a bid to provide lasting solutions in the areas of health and life longevity, this book becomes an essential vade mecum for both model researchers, or those working practically as healthcare practitioners, as well as people striving for improvement of their lifespan.

Through deciphering the molecular mechanisms, therapeutic efficacy, and adverse effects of every drug in use, Longevity delivers a two-sided read about the positives and negatives associated with pharmacologic intervention to aging. The book is effective at doing this and by its careful analysis, provides the reader with essential information necessary for right decisions on whether or not to fight old age.

There is a need to define the innate transformative nature of age-related pharmacological intervention, which at first glance seems as a new horizon for healthcare today where longevity and productivity are potential. For the continuously progressing longevity science, "Longevity" is a source of knowledge and an efficient guide to navigate in the rapidly developing maze of aging.

Finally, this book becomes a master work in the field of mortality discourse whereby it is seen as an important shift in perception that highlights aging and life. By drawing on a systematic combination of empirical data, clinical wisdom and creative vista, the book contributes not only to making clear the path towards extended longevity but also to enable readers to assert command over their own functional journeys viably leading towards vitality. By accomplishing this, it initiates a paradigm change calling people to proactively participate in the perpetual saga of human mortality by way of educated decisions and discovery of agency.

1.2. Understanding Aging and Health in Contemporary Society

For a suitable aging and health understanding, which is especially relevant in the rapidly changing world of modern society. In light of the rapid developments in science and medicine that both help expand human life, a clear understanding of how aging occurs becomes apparent along with maintaining an optimal health at all stages of life can no longer be dismissed as irrelevant. And this investigation in depth and shed light on the multi-layered causes of realizing the importance of aging and health in contemporary society.

a) **Addressing Demographic Shifts**

In the modern world of global community, changing demographics are altering at an unconventional rate and significantly characterized by a growing number elderly people within people. This evolution illustrates a wider demographic transition that is defined by diminishing birth rates despite the numbers of people living up to longer ages. Such a significant transformation of population dynamics completely reinstructs the social tissue presenting wide-ranging threats and vulnerabilities encompassing virtually every sphere, in particular, health care, systems of interaction and economics.

The latter is characterized by the necessity to understand aging in its multilayered manifestations. Aging is not strictly physical; instead, it can be described as a compounded progressive interaction of the physiological, psychological and social dimensions. In a physiological way, aging means the slow weakening of functions and resistance of body parts such that people become more prone to chronic diseases and disabilities. Psychologically, aging behavior may include cognitive changes, emotional adjustments and existential reflections to understand life stages. In the social sense of things, aging at the family level is impacted by familial relationships, community dynamics as well as societal norms and all these contribute to inclusionary experiences, support networks as well as fulfillment.

This trend of growing elderly populations highlights the urgent need for personalised approaches to meet specific requirements and challenges that are innate to aging processes and health. For instance, healthcare systems are required to adjust to changing demographic trends through a shift of services provision with an emphasis on the need for geriatric care, pre-emptive interventions and management of chronic diseases It entails investments in health care infrastructure investment, human resources development amid research initiatives aimed to quality-of-life improvement and healthy aging advancement across lifespans.

Furthermore, the impacts of demographic changes encompass more than health care and affect broader social architecture and economic models. Families develop into new forms due to the modification of intergenerational support and accommodation networks, which alter their traditional shapes according to the changes in demographics and socio-cultural values. Women are usually the primary caregiver, which adds to the caregiving burden incurred by women and emphasizes a need for gender-sensitive policies and social support programs focused on alleviating strain that is caused by caregiving responsibilities.

Moreover, this economic impacting of the aging people is felt within other sectors such as labor markets, pension programmes and fiscal policies of every country. However, demographic dividend, once received as the driver of economic growth and development, now extends fiscal implications towards social security systems and pension funds provided to aging population. Achieving the fiscal sustainability of social welfare relies implicitly on innovation to balance equity, responsibility and cohesion between generations.

In responding to the demographic changes, policymakers, researchers, and practitioners must find multidimensional approaches that cross disciplinary borders encompassing diversity among aging experiences. The impact of interdisciplinary collaboration in promoting innovation that centralizes on supporting healthy aging, social inclusion, and reducing the gap among elderly population is inevitable. This involves developing collaboration between healthcare institutions, social service agencies, educational establishments and community centers to capitalize on the diverse skills and resources necessary for addressing the comprehensive needs of an aging population.

Similarly, creating age-friendly settings that support active aging and ensure older adulthood is still active, integrated in personal life through health outcome enhancement and quality of life across the entire lifespan. This includes constructing those built environments that are accessible, advocating for age friendly policies and encouraging intergenerational cohesion to build communities, where all ages feel at home.

b) **Promoting Healthy Aging**

Aging is a complex journey that everyone takes through numerous physical and psychological changes and the social aspect of change. The process of aging is considered natural and unavoidable; however, the well-being in this period can be dramatically improved by preventative actions associated with promoting healthy ageing. This investigation, therefore, reveals the complexities of healthy ageing including the interaction between personal decision-making, clinical interventions and community settings in fostering positive wellness as individuals age along the venerable phase of life.

- Understanding Healthy Aging:

The basis of healthy aging, therefore, can simply be defined as a practice that is comprehensive and goes beyond mere lack of illness to incorporate physical wellbeing, satisfaction. It involves improving various body systems, maintaining mental sharpness, developing the ability to bounce back after emotional adversities and building bonds. There are many aspects that influence health aging including genes, family factors or backgrounds that may affect the life itself.

- Lifestyle Choices and Healthy Aging:

Self-empowerment is one of the main components inherent to healthy aging and consists in people making their lifetime choices that ensure both energy and long life. Developing healthy sleep patterns, eating a balanced diet containing adequate nutrients, and engaging in physical activity on a daily basis are the cornerstones of successful aging. Aerobic exercise enables to maintain muscle, strengthens bones and optimize cardiovascular state, as well as has positive impacts on the cognitive performance. Similarly, a nutritionally dense diet of whole fruits and vegetables, whole grains, and lean meats are high in those same growth promoting nutrients that maintain cellular function. In addition, developing interests, practicing and attending to learning through the lifespan along with maintaining activities from gratifying social interaction also help provide stimulation for the sustenance of cognition and enjoyment leading to a purposeful life.

- <u>Healthcare Interventions in Healthy Aging:</u>

High-performing healthcare interventions provide a crucial link to achieving healthy aging as they prevent, diagnose and manage GERD comorbidities. Preventive care measures like health screening programs, vaccinations and health education campaign on lifestyle helps individuals to act early when they are faced with health problems. The recycled paper feeds into the university's Ecology Program by showcasing its commitment to environmental conservation. In addition, disease management interventions geared toward the geriatric population attenuate the physical effects of chronic medical issues like diabetes arthritis and hypertension all these factors cumulatively improve quality of life and also promote functional autonomy. Similarly, patients require broad availability of comprehensive geriatric care resources such as geriatric assessment, medication management, and caregiver assistance in addition to addressing the multiple medical requirements for a general population that is aging.

c) **<u>Mitigating the Burden of Age-Related Diseases</u>**

Age-related illnesses continue to pose a daunting threat on the contemporary medical settings, with both individuals and infrastructure turning insurmountably heavy. The conditions include cardiovascular complications, neuro- related illnesses, and even metabolic syndromes not only make the quality of life sickening for affected persons but weaken health care systems around the world. It becomes vitally necessary to venture into the insides of how these intricacies are guided by distinct mechanisms that define such diseases in relation to ageing. However, only with a holistic understanding of disease's origins and progression at the genetic level as well as then lifestyle factors and environmental influences upon disease onset and development can researchers reveal novel paths for intervention and prevention thus completely redefining ageing paradigm.

Thus, hidden in the depth of mitigating age-related diseases are many secrets with regard to deciphering how heredity and environment interact. Even though gene predispositions might play a part in laying the ground for many age-related conditions susceptibility, factorials from environment usually come up as catalysts igniting when environmental factors escalate disease processes. Analysing the delicate dance by these factors makes it possible to determine main molecular pathways involved in disease development. In an example, the discovery of variant prone to cardiovascular diseases has led to treatment on targets signaling pathway thus controlling disease progression in high-risk population.

Additionally, lifestyle factors have great influence of the occurrence and course of various age-related diseases. Sedentary lifestyle, nutritional choices, and tobacco exhibited are non-modifiable risk factors on which takes up a significant burden is spread across different population groups of nations. Industrial initiatives as well as educational campaigns give individuals a chance to adopt healthier lifestyles, thus lowering the possibility of developing age-related diseases. In addition, the progress has been made in digital health technologies that allow monitoring of lifestyle metrics and individual approaches to cultured special interventions that meet specific need and preference.

Parallel to genetic and lifestyle factors, environmental impacts play a vital part of the disease's nature. In the presence of environmental chemicals, pollutants, and oxidative poly-suppressors exposure can cause cellular injury and inflammatory responses creating an environment suitable for development of age-related pathology. The molecular mechanisms by which environmental factors bring about changes are the key to enabling scientists to develop ways of preventing their impact that is harmful to human health. From specific antioxidant interventions to environment preservation strategies, multi directional measures should be taken to protect subjects from the harm caused by environmental agents.

At the center of efforts geared towards age-related disease control are research and development initiatives aimed at finding novel therapeutic regimens designed to address underlying causes of pathology. In terms of therapies against age-related disorders, small molecule inhibitors of aberrant pathways that target specific molecular processes or gene editing technologies have significantly improved in the past decade to correct genetic mutations. What is more, with the emergence of regenerative medicine, not only one can restore the function of tissues but also reverse aging process bringing new hope into life for patients suffering from degenerative diseases.

In this regard, together with therapeutic interventions a proactive approach to disease prevention is crucial for reducing the commitment of age-related diseases. In addition to early detection screenings, risk stratification algorithms, and personalized prevention plans is an opportunity for people to safeguard health even in old age. In addition, the blending of predictive analytics and artificial intelligence could also enable detection of high-risk individuals whose interventions can be designed to their individual uniqueness making the prevention strategies highly effective.

d) <u>Addressing Healthcare Inequities</u>

The health care disparity that persistently lingers in the contemporary society only leaves an indelible mark on the public health fabric. This is evident on the fact that people in different categories of race and ethnicities, poor social economic classes, as well as minority groups are all discriminated when it comes to receiving health care services. These inequities not only undermine the fundamental principles of justice and equity but also create formidable obstacles to optimal health for all concern individuals.

This multilayered issue is at its core the need to understand seniority and health from the lenses of equity and social justice. Indeed, by clarifying the complex dynamic interactions between factors at societal and economic levels, as well as structural biases, healthcare inequalities can be more comprehensively addressed.

Acknowledgment that health is a critical element of the human right is at the heart of the pursuit of health equity. However, as a society in the age of tremendous medical progress and technology, we should tear down structural hurdles that limit the provision of crucial health care services. Either by the expanding healthcare coverage, setting up community-based clinics in areas that are lacking facilities and services or through provision of culturally sensitive care people need to make concerted efforts in ensuring universal accessibility and responsiveness to concentrated needs in diverse populations.

In addition, the necessity to eliminate health disparities does not stop at access but extends to issues of quality and cultural competency. Systemic prejudices and discriminatory policies are found in many healthcare settings, which leads to the poor outcome of treatment for people from marginalized groups that only worsen health disparities. In an effort to reduce these differences, health care providers have to go through intense training in cultural competency and implicit bias recognition so that they can deliver patient-centered care sensitive of the individual needs and preferences associated with a diverse patient population.

Besides tackling issues of unequally distributed access to and quality of healthcare, health equity efforts should also include a general preventative care and promote the concept of holistic health. By promoting preventative methods, early detection, and health education programmes in disadvantaged areas of society can create a more proactive attitude among individuals to protect their health and livelihood. These interventions have a vital role to play in advancing health literacy, promoting lifestyle changes and reducing disparities on preventable diseases across diverse populations.

e) <u>Informing Policy and Resource Allocation</u>

Policy makers move through a terrain beset by multidimensional issues ranging from demography to needs for infrastructure for health. A multitude of resources, such as strong facts, academic literature and specialized professionals are used by them to weather this complicated landscape. These inputs provide policymakers with the knowledge required to design regulatorily systems, allocate financial resources wisely and properly formulate programs specifically targeted at specific age groups.

Interdisciplinary collaboration becomes an indispensable enabler in formulating overall policy resolutions. By bringing in multidimensional insights gathered from a variety of fields like medicine, public health, economics and social sciences policymakers can come up with comprehensive strategies that can deal with the complicated dynamics behind aging. An integrated strategy allows policy makers to address the cumulative complexities presented by an older society—from health care availability to inequitable socioeconomic status.

In addition, a sophisticated understanding of aging and health foments constructive practices in the form of healthy aging options. Through the establishment of enabling environment that promote wellness and preventive approach, policymakers seek to suppress the occurrence of age-related pathologies as well as increase quality life standards for elderly individuals. By implementing select interventions around health education, community participation, and lifestyle management policies aimed at improving the quality of the life for aging populations.

Essentially, the informing of policy and resource allocation requires a joint effort to make decisions that are evidence-based, involve interdisciplinary collaboration and continuous engagement with the fast-changing needs of aging populations. Yet when policymakers internalize these values, they are transformed into agents who can untangle the web of challenges brought about by an aging society with precision, compassion and far-sightedness for societal well being.

1.3.   Preview of the book's structure and content

In this book, the readers embark on a generalized sought after aging, health and longevity. Through this book, a multi-dimensional approach is provided towards the intricate nature of interactions between lifestyle preferences and pharmacological intervention with emphasis on emerging advanced technology modulations for longevity and vitality.

- <u>Understanding Aging and Health</u>

The first chapters of the book allow for an understanding of aging and health at a basic level. In this, readers examine the complex biological mechanisms involved in aging and learn about various processes whose involvement is significant like cell senescence, oxidative stress and genomic instabilities. Through this clarification, readers understand better their significance via proactive management of health and how they may be intervened.

- <u>Exploring Lifestyle Practices for Longevity</u>

More than ones of the book focus on life-style practice that leads to long life and vigor. The sub-chapters target on nutrition, exercise, management of stressful conditions and sleep that play crucial roles in preserving a healthy life during aging. The readers, acquire knowledge on the physiological impact of nutrition, gains from consistent physical activity and means for managing stress and the importance of proper sleep in meeting overall well-being. Readers are equipped with practical guidelines and actionable advice, enabling them to implement these lifestyle practices into their everyday lives and promoting a self-determined approach to health enhancement.

- Untangling the Working of Age Prolonging Drugs

Another thematic focus of the book is a search for longevity drugs in particular Rapamycin, Metformin and Acarbose. The readers are given in-depth analysis of cellular and molecular mechanisms which the medications employ to produce their effect. For instance, the way in which Rapamycin suppresses the mTOR pathway emulates the results of restricted caloric intake, whilst Metformin's activation of AMPK improves cellular energy efficiency. The book clarifies how these drugs act in a finer mechanism and control metabolism, reduce inflammatory processes, as well as prevent oxidative stress to improve longevity and health span.

- Evaluating Pharmacological Approaches to Longevity

In subsequent chapters, the book provides a critical assessment of potential advantages and disadvantages that would result from pharmacological interventions which aim at increasing longevity. By using scientific discoveries and clinical evidence, readers are given a glimpse into the effectiveness, safety and ethical issues related to anti-aging medication use. By means of balanced debate, the book promotes a prudent consideration of the pros and cons of pharmacological interventions that will enable sound decisions with health care practitioners.

- **In addition to the Future of Aging and Health.**

As the book comes towards its conclusion, readers are encouraged to reflect on the wider ethical dilemmas that longevity science presents for personal and societal relationships alongside issues surrounding how healthcare systems manage longevity. Topics of the discussion include moral problems and prevailing attitudes towards elderly people, as well as require fair provision of healthcare interventions. Through positioning longevity within a wider societal and ethical perspective, the book inspires readers envision a more comprehensive vision of the future that comprises advanced life spans together with improved popularity along with aftermath.

CHAPTER 2
UNDERSTANDING AGING AND HEALTH

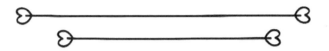

2.1. The Biology of Aging: Key Processes and Mechanisms

C larifying the biology of aging is an important step to unveiling the puzzles associated with human aging length and strategies for healthy-aging promotion. Human aging is a complex multifactorial process that involves many genetic, environmental, and lifestyle factors. In this discussion, we attempt to explain the core processes and mechanisms of aging wherein tightly regulated cellular and molecular processes fully unfold.

a) Cellular Senescence: A Hallmark of Aging

There is an important feature of the aging process hidden in the complex pattern of cellular senescence, which includes dissociation with a cell division and subsequent damage to the function. Age-related atrophy of LPS represents a hallmark feature of aging present across different tissues and organisms, significantly affecting the whole physiology and health span in individuals. Elucidating the mechanisms and implications of cellular senescence is fundamental for understanding ageing, as well as preventing or treating various degenerative diseases caused by this phenomenon.

Cellular senescence roots deepness in molecular events, which is predetermined by a multitude of factors. Widespread, persistent DNA damage is one of the main factors that contribute to cellular senescence. This DNA damage accumulates with aging due to exposure to various environmental stresses, endogenous metabolism and other intrinsic and extrinsic factors. The reparation of DNA lesions is one characteristic that gradually lowers in cells as they age which causes the activation of some signaling pathways, leading to cellular senescence.

Another major mechanism propelling cellular senescence is the process of telomere shortening. During cell division there is shortening in the lengths of individual telomeres as protective caps are to form at the end. Eventually, with them being too critical, telomeres activate a DNA damage response that makes cells senescent as an emergency mechanism against genomic instability and malignancy.

Oxidative stress, which is attributable to the disproportionation of ROS production and antioxidant defenses, is also a major factor that can induce cellular senescence. A significant source of damage in cells caused by the activity of ROS includes DNA, proteins and lipids which initiate pathways leading to senescence hence contributes to aging.

Cellular senescence impacts tissue homeostasis and organismal fitness by effects more than just the individual cell. Senescent cells release a broad sheet of bioactive molecules in aggregate known as the senescence-associated secretory phenotype (SASP). The SASP includes various pro-inflammatory cytokines, growth factors, proteases and other ligands that shape the tissue microenvironment as well as neighborhood cells. The main functions of the SASP are to serve as a reaction on the stress stimulus and to promote the tissue repair and regeneration at first; however, all chronic secretion of SASP components by senescent cells can lead to a long-lasting inflammation with pathology development.

Cellular senescence can thus be considered a pivotal landmark of the aging process depriving the cells of proliferation and vitality. It is the complicated reciprocity of DNA damage, telomere shortening, oxidative stress and others what underlies the incipient and perpetuation of senescence cellular pathways. To elucidate the mechanisms and dynamics of aging, it is important to understand cellular senescence and its effects in order to help create interventions for healthy aging and treatment of age-related diseases.

b) <u>Telomere Attrition and Cellular Aging</u>

Telomeres gain the status of crucial shields of genome integrity and de facto judges of cellular destiny. These tiny structures that lurk at the ends of chromosomes serve as 'sentinels' warding off the blights of time and the continual assaults posed by cell proliferation. Telomeres made up of repetitive DNA sequences attached to the chromosome by specialized proteins serve as a guard against degradation and fusion therefore ensuring normalcy of the genomic integrity.

Unyielding cell division leads to constant shortening of telomeres, a phenomenon that is termed telomere attrition. This is because each cycle of replication leads to the occurrence of the process referred as end-replication problem in which DNA polymerases cannot copy terminal regions on linear chromosomes. As a result, telomeres undergo progressive erosion, approaching irreparably that fatal threshold which signals senescence or apoptosis.

The rate of telomere shortening is not solely controlled by the inner mechanism of cellular replication but depends broadly on a large number of extrinsic factors. Chronic stress is an inevitable phantom in contemporary living, which causes a prolonged physiological load, leading to the chain reaction of hormonal and immunologic effects accelerating telomere shortening. In addition, the chronic low-grade inflammation that is an accompaniment of aging driven by a milieu of pro-inflammatory cytokines and oxidative stress conspires to wear away at the telomeric integrity contributing to accelerated age on cellular level.

Of great insidiousness is oxidative damage due to reactive oxygen species which are generated during normal cellular metabolism. The guanine-rich sequences in telomeric DNA are also vulnerable to oxidative harm of the type that results in DNA lesions and strand breaks impairing their integrity and functionality, leading to the rapid attrition.

Besides, new research points to the role of lifestyle factors like nutrition, physical activity and social interactivity in shaping the rate at which telomeres shorten highlighting the complex interplay between genotype and environment as determinants of cellular aging patterns.

Telomere shortening remains a telltale sign of cellular senescence—a systemic erosion of the very foundation by which genomic integrity rests leading to inevitable senescence. The deciphering molecular pathways relevant to telomere regulation reveals entirely new ways of intervention, which promote the exciting opportunities that lie ahead in terms of combating age-related diseases and achieving longevity. As a result, the pursuit of this understanding of telomere biology marks an epochal change in our views on aging and gives visions into a tomorrow where the age-old dictate of time may be softened with molecular knowledge.

c) <u>Mitochondrial Dysfunction: Impact on Aging</u>

Mitochondria are the true work horses of eukaryotic cells that serve as the essential centers for cellular energetics and metabolism. The function of these organelles is the manufacturing of adenosine triphosphate (ATP), which serves as the primary energy currency for cells to carry out other biochemical processes required for life to continue. Yet, despite the crucial role that mitochondria play in organisms' cells, with age these structures undergo progressive degradation known as mitochondrial dysfunction.

The heart of mitochondrial dysfunction is the reduction in mitochondrial energy passage, which results from reduced electron transport chain (ETC) function. Mitochondria also grow old with age so that ATP synthesis becomes less effective and cellular energy levels drop as a consequence. At the same time, mitochondria, which are dysfunctional feature an enhanced tendency to produce ROS as products of oxidative phosphorylation. Yet, there are ROS such as superoxide anions and hydrogen peroxide acting like double-edged swords; they contribute to normal physiological signaling pathways but excessive ROS production overcomes the ability of the endogenous antioxidant defenses leading to oxidative damage at cellular macromolecules.

Mitochondrial faults that contribute to ATP insufficiency and oxidative stress have other destructive effects. The occurrence of accumulated oxidized and dysfunctional mitochondria, able to maintain optimal respiratory function, activates a series of adverse processes that affect the integrity and cellular homeostasis. It displaces intermediary metabolic pathways leading to the disruptions of these nutrients. In addition, the mitochondrial dysfunction disrupts calcium homeostasis and leads to shifting cellular signaling cascades towards apoptotic death.

Interestingly, the effects of mitochondrial damage are, however, not only limited to the intra-cellular environment but spread across organ systems playing a pivotal role in disease development of a range of age related disorders. Neurodegenerative disorders, such as Alzheimer and Parkinson's are diseases defined by considerably progressive shrinkage of neurons that is intrinsically linked to mitochondrial dysfunctional and oxidative stress-mediated reduction in bioenergetic functions.

Also, mitochondrial dysfunctions- associated reduction in myocardial contractility and vascular endothelial dysfunction intensifies cardiac pathologies such as heart failure atherosclerosis. Metabolic syndromes, which include obesity, type 2 diabetes and insulin resistance disorders are initiated due to disequilibrium of mitochondrial energetics, problems with glucose and lipid biochemistry.

d) <u>Inflammation and Immunosenescence</u>

Immune senescence and associated phenomena of inflammation are highly relevant, especially for the process of aging and age-related disorders. Chronic low-grade inflammation or as it is known, "inflammaging," appears to be one of the distinguishing marks of aging and this process becomes intertwined with many physiological systems.

Immunosenescence or the abnormal behavior of the immune system during age serves as a primary companion to inflammaging. Through ageing, the immune system goes through a series of changes in its development which modifies their landscape of immune cell composition, functionality and signaling cascades. Such changes, while seemingly minor, have tremendous powers in the body's capacity to conduct viable immune responses against pathogens and malignant cells.

These repercussions of immunosenescence echo across the physical body ending in more intense inflammatory reactions and immune weakened state. The destruction of the fine balance between immune surveillance and response mechanisms leaves them susceptible to various pathologies among aged individuals.

Infections are perhaps some of the most touching effects of immunosenescence, as the immune system begins to weaken and fail to contribute significant defense against invading disease-causing organisms. Further, the detailed protocols that support self-tolerance collapse leading to autoimmune diseases through which the immune system attacks its own tissues.

Equally, cancer is presented as a ghost coming from the horizon taking advantage of the vulnerabilities of retired immunosenescent defense Due to the weakening of the immune system's capacity to eradicate malignant cells and growing without restriction, cancer tissues are made even more uncomfortable.

the intersection of inflammation and Immunosenescence forms an interlinkage inescapably associated with time. The crucial element of this understanding is the depth penetration which allows revealing possible therapeutic channels that can help to cope with aging and strengthening immunity elsewhere.

e) Epigenetic Alterations: Modulating Gene Expression

Epigenetic changes including DNA methylation, histone modifications and the regulation of non-coding RNAs form a diverse regulatory framework; they direct the expression patterns and identity of cells. These changes act on factors other than the DNA sequence, in constantly changing both processes and gene activity, and phenotypic results. But the epigenetic landscape is not stable and goes through dramatic changes within aging involved in determines transcriptional patterns and cellular responses.

Among the major mechanisms leading to epigenetic alterations are DNA methylation based on covalent attachment of methyl group to cytosine residues linked in CpG dinucleotides. In the process of aging, dramatic remodeling in the DNA methylation patterns takes place that brings about significant global alterations in expression from different cell types and tissues. The histone modifications, which include acetylation methylation phosphorylation and ubiquitination also adds to the complexity of the chromatin's regulation structure and accessibility. During aging, errant histone modifications lead to the disruption of homeostasis in gene activation and suppression that weakens cellular functions.

Apart from coding RNAs, noncoding RNAs such as microRNAs, long noncoding RNAs and circular RNA also contribute to epigenetic regulation by influencing mRNA stability and translation efficiency. Imbalance of non-coding RNAs in the aging does not keep equilibrium of gene expression networks, disrupting cellular homeostasis and provoking the pathogenesis.

In combination, age-related changes in epigenetic factors give rise to cellular dysfunction and genomic instability, which is associated with an increased likelihood of developing a wide variety of age-related disorders including cancer, neurodegenerative disorders, and metabolic syndromes. The disruption of core epigenetic processes highlights the complex interplay between genetic predisposition and through environmental hookups in dictating how health trajectories unroll over the lifespan.

The elucidation of the complicated interactions between epigenetic modifications and aging represents a significant therapeutic implication that provides exceptional potential for treating age-related pathologies. Such precise targeting of particular epigenetic regulators might propose a potential approach for changing age-related epigenetic changes, resolving cellular equilibrium, as well as increasing health span in aging populations.

Thus, elucidating the intricate complexities of epigenetic modulation represents a crucial endeavor in the pursuit of healthier aging and enhanced quality of life.

f) <u>Hormonal Changes and Aging</u>

The human body, with age, undergoes a chain of complicated psychophysical transformations influenced by hormonal changes. Hormones act as vital agents of communication, controlling many physiological processes starting from growth and metabolism to reproduction and cognition. However, aging undermines the precision of these hormonal signaling pathways leading to a sequence of events that involve different tissues in the body.

The hormonal changes that are most remarkable in the aging process include reduced production of major hormones like estrogen, testosterone, and growth hormone. Estrone, the main component of estrogen best known for its contributions to reproductive health and bone density has diminished in postmenopausal women resulting from increased risk of osteoporosis, and cardiovascular events. Indeed, the levels of testosterones reduce gradually in men affecting muscle mass, libido as well as vitality. Some of the hormones that decline with age include Growth Hormone which is essential to tissue repair and muscle growth thus contributing towards weakening muscles strength, slower wound healing process.

Such hormonal changes do not only affect reproductive endocrines, but they are extended to the larger endocrine network and affect insulin sensitivity, thyroid function, and stress response. Dysregulation of insulin and glucose metabolism will make people susceptible to diabetes, Changes in thyroid hormones may result in weight gain, fatigue as well impaired cognition. In addition, alterations in HPA can lead to improper stress management that leads to depression and anxiety as age-related problems.

In addition, hormone-aging interaction is not limited to physical health only; it also affects neurocognitive mechanisms as well as mental state. For example, estrogen has neuroprotective properties in the brain and its deficiency is related to age-related cognitive decline seen with increased risk of developing neurodegenerative diseases like Alzheimer's disease. Testosterone is also involved in cognitive functions, promoting spatial skills and memory performance as well as regulating mood.

2.2.   Impact of Lifestyle on Longevity and Vitality

Lifestyle is an essential component in the mission for long life and bliss. Our lifestyle – food, sport, stress-control as well as sleeping patterns and other choice of our routines plays a very important role in determining our overall health condition. This section depicts the various complexities of lifestyle as a factor behind longevity and vitality, factoring in such details, as the relationship between physiology mechanisms and lifestyle choices.

a) Diet and Nutrition

Food and nutrition are a sovereign pillar to human life which lays the essence of living forever. The importance of adopting a healthy and balanced diet cannot be overemphasized, as such practices are at the center of promoting well-being across generations by reducing the prevalence and threat of chronic conditions. Research strongly emphasizes the fact that food choices have a significant role in determining one's health and therefore, emphasis should be placed on pursuing an ideal dietary regime rich in many nutrients.

First and foremost, foods rich in essential nutrients such as vitamins, minerals, antioxidants and phytochemicals should be the core of a healthy diet meal. The basic materials for a healthy diet include fruits, vegetables, whole grains as well as lean proteins and healthier fats, which are essential to fuel the body and supply all the required nutrients. Antioxidant-rich foods such as berries and leafy greens can be seen to boost oxidative stress that is related to aging and disease development in a very complex way.

The Mediterranean diet, an example of a healthy-eating pattern linked to decreased risk for cardiovascular comorbidity and favorable effects on life expectancy, emphasizes vegetarian foods, lean proteins and olive oil. This commitment to promoting whole, minimally processed foods also captured the importance of adopting dietary practices harmonious with natural and nutrient-rich origins.

On the other hand, high consumption of processed foods, refined sugars and saturated fats carries grave health implications. Such lifestyles promote inflammation, insulin resistance and free-radical damage leading to premature aging with increasing risk of various age related conditions.

The realization of how nutritional food choices play a critical role in one's health highlights the need to be deliberate and also choose right types of diets. The development of nutritional habits contributing to the prolonged life and vitality requires a purposeful attitude to choices of foods, focusing on natural food rich in nutrients and avoiding any processed foods with much sugar.

By embracing a nourishing diet replete with wholesome foods, individuals can pave the way toward optimal health and well-being, fostering a foundation for vitality and resilience across the lifespan.

b) **Exercise and Physical Activity**

With the goal of a dynamic and lasting life, regular physical exercise naturally appears as one basis, holding all potential physiological and psychological perks. Exercise, instead of a simple and generic process, is the determinant of how long one lives in good condition.

Exercise is the agent of transformation that triggers physiological change. Aerobic exercises, like brisk walking, running or swimming since they bring about a concert of cardiovascular improvements. They manage to lure the heart into a well organized beat, increasing circulation, reducing blood pressure and strengthening the body's resistance against cardiovascular disorder. By participating regularly in aerobic physical activity, individuals attain a strong cardiovascular system that stands up the ordeals of aging and the siege of chronic illnesses.

However, the landscape of physical activity extends beyond that of aerobic effort. Resistance training comes out as a tough competitor for the body-building exercise and the buildup of its infrastructure. Whether through the clanging of pounding weights or slowing body resistance against gravity, the muscles are pushed to development, benefits increased bone mass and helps musculature survives enemy of age. This symphony of strength builds a barrier against the aging process, and people stand firm as shakes turn into ages.

Nevertheless, the rewards of workouts stretch much beyond the physical spheres. The mind takes its long vacation in the heat of exertion. With exercise comes an antidote for the spirit of weariness; a remedy that heals the wounds caused by stress anxiety, depression. With each harmony of movement, peoples find a sanctuary of peace, an oasis on which the drudgeries of life dissipate into thin air. In addition, exercising enhances cognitive activity cultivating brain networks that glow with bright intention, lighting the hallways of the mind with the dazzling effulgence of life.

Then, it seems that the exercise is one of the threads that connect fabric of health and happiness. It is a symbol to the perseverance of mankind which shines amidst the tempestuous waves of life. The power of transformation becomes individuals' road to find themselves, step by step trying to make light with the setting whatever makes him healthy and alive. Therefore, let us accept the gift of exercise and in its arms start to reveal unlimited opportunities we have inside ourselves.

c) <u>Stress Management</u>

Chronic stress can now be seen as a powerful enemy to the overall well-being, targeting the physical and mental health functions. Chronic stress is a state of constant exposure to stressors, and it causes physiological alterations that can significantly impact the body and mind. Ill effects of stress, from increased levels of cortisol to systemic inflammation are far-reaching and long lasting.

Among the forefronts of stress management is its demeanor in relation to how it undermines life span and vitality. Chronic stress not only impairs the immune system but it accelerates premature cellular aging and establishes the ground for a plethora of chronic diseases such as cardiovascular diseases, diabetes, and neurodegenerative disorders. The necessity of dealing with stress as one of the causes for the decline of health cannot be exaggerated.

Stress management techniques involve a variety of coping mechanisms aimed at alleviating the devastating impacts of stress and enhancing the ability to remain steadfast in adverse situations. From these approaches, mindfulness practice turns into a light in the middle of darkness and gives practitioners an escape point from the turmoil of life. Through the promotion of presence and mindful acceptance, mindfulness meditation halts the malaise cycle, enabling one to respond to stress with a greater degree of equanimity.

The deep breathing exercises that form another pillar of stress management take advantage of the breath to cause relaxation and create an atmosphere where the balance between the autonomic nervous system is restored. By breathing intentionally and diaphragmatically, individuals can put the parasympathetic response into action, overriding stress-connected physiological arousal.

With fusion of movement, breath and mindfulness together yoga provides a global approach to stress management. As a result of coordinating the body and mind through a sequence of postures and breathing exercises, yoga generates strength of body, clarity in the mind, and endurance to stay calm. By moving through poses with intention, the practitioners are able to maintain a high level of awareness in each pose building a sense of presence that transcends their stress-based reactiveness.

Besides the organized practices such as meditations and yoga, recreation constitute some of the effectual antidotes to stress. Whether it's enjoying the great outdoors, practicing art and other creative pastimes, or bonding with friends and loved ones, they are important to relax the mind from the demands of every day life.

For certain, stress management is more than just relieving symptoms but about creating a life that embodies balance, durability and vigour. With mindfulness, deep breathing, yoga and leisure pursuits, people can strengthen themselves against the ill-will of malicious stress leaving a residual fight for survival. Despite the fact that life is a series of inevitable challenges, the practice of stress control techniques provides an avenue to perpetual vitality and blossoming.

d) <u>Sleep Hygiene</u>

Sleep hygiene is collective name for the range of practices and habits aimed at encouraging healthy, restorative sleeping patterns. Such approaches are essential to improving sleep quality and duration, which allows for proper function of the body as a whole being.

Establishing a regular sleep pattern remains one of the essential aspects of proper sleep hygiene. The body's internal clock, which is measured as circadian rhythm, regulated through similar sleeping and waking times even on weekends. This routine helps to support the natural circadian cycle of the body thereby making it easier to fall asleep and wake up feeling refreshed.

Another important characteristic of sleep hygiene is ensuring that the surrounding environment promotes sleep. It is desirable that the sleep environment be homely, soft and free of noises. This might include purchasing a soft mattress and cushions, maintaining the room's temperature moderately cool, and eliminating noise sources to reduce disruptions. Furthermore, the exposure to blue light emitted from electronic devices like smartphones, tablets and laptops disrupts the natural production of melatonin hormone which is responsible for sleep regulation. By minimizing the amount of time people spend on screens before bed can help minimize this disturbance and get a better quality sleep.

Relaxation techniques are also good for sleep hygiene even before sleeping. Activities that will calm the mind and body effectively include meditation, deep breathing exercises, gentle stretching. By avoiding arousing activities like strenuous exercise and ingesting caffeine or nicotine just before sleep, calmness is aided, and the quality of one's sleep improves.

In addition, leading a healthy life is critical in promoting optimal sleep hygiene. Daytime's physical activity can help encourage deep and restful sleep at night. Yet it is recommended not to engage in a workout just before going to sleep, as this can lead to fettering and impede the sleeping process. The same applies to taking heavy meals, alcohol, and stimulants during evening hours because they disturb the sleep cycles.

Sleep hygiene should, therefore, not be overlooked when it comes to promoting total health. Consistent sleep schedules, making the environment conducive to rest, relaxation activities and positive life practices can ensure optimal quality of sleep and its prolongation. Through such action, they can enjoy the multitude of benefits that sleep restores; better cognition, mood regulation and immunity this ensures longevity and vitality.

2.3. The Concept of Pharmacological Approaches to Longevity

In the process of striving to lengthen human lifespan, such researchers and medical practitioners have shifted more into pharmacological methods. These approaches involve the administration of drugs and compounds that target biological pathways associated with age, to aim at slowing aging processes while improving overall well-being. Pharmacological interventions in longevity signifies a remarkable frontier within medical science that presents opportunities for meeting the obstacles of population ageing and promoting quality of life standards for individuals around the globe.

a) **Understanding the Aging Process**

In order to create successful methods of achieving longevity and preventing age-related diseases, the aging process should be understood. However, old age is not just the passing of time but a complicated biologic process characterized by a diminution of physiological function and susceptibility to many diseases. In order to investigate possible pharmacological interventions for the development of therapies aimed at potentially enhancing lifespan, it is necessary to understand mechanisms underlying aging.

The ageing phenomenon is powered by many interdependent factors, both intracellular and systemic. Genomic instability, one of the fundamental features of aging, includes accumulation of DNA damage during time that carries with it errors in genetic information and a violation of the cell function. Another significant aspect of aging is telomere shortening, which entails the gradual wear down of protective covers at the conclusion of chromosomes that are related to cellular senescence and genomic unsteadiness.

Epigenetic modifications, such as DNA methylation of histone modification, act centrally in controlling gene expression and altering cell function throughout the aging process. The insufficient proteostatic balance leading to the disordered protein synthesis and degradation contributes to the accumulation of misfolded proteins that are characteristic for age-related neurodegenerative disorders such as Alzheimer's and Parkinson's disease.

Mitochondrial dysfunction, which accompanies the process of aging and reflects its properties is characterized by reduced energy production and increased oxidative penetration. It is well known that cellular senescence that involves in the extensive unresponsive arrest of cell proliferation due to different stimuli, particularly contributes tissue decay and chronic inflammation, giving rise to disease progression in age-related diseases.

In addition, deregulated nutrient sensing pathways including dull-like insulin/insulin-like growth factor 1 (IGF-1) signaling pathway regulate metabolic homeostasis and lifespan in different organisms ranging from yeast to mammals. The impairment of these pathways can accelerate ageing and render a person metabolic disease such as diabetes and obesity.

Aging is multi-layered choreographed by a system of interconnected molecular and cellular states. Although the exact biological pathways underlying aging are yet to be fully understood, research has pinpointed genomic instability, telomere shortening, epigenetic modifications, proteostasis disruption, mitochondrial impairment, cellular senescence and nutrient sensing deregulation as principal driving forces of the aging phenotype. Through a detailed understanding of these underlying mechanisms, scientists can use pharmacological interventions that target the healthy aging of people and prolonging their lifespan.

b) <u>Rationale for Pharmacological Interventions</u>

As an avenue in the search for a medicine to expand human lifespan, pharmacological interventions are grounded on an advanced interpretation of aging as a multi-dimensional biological process. But aging is not a passive end product of time; it is now conceptualized as the net result of molecular and cellular interactions within an organism. The researchers investigating longevity assume that these mechanisms are adjustable and therefore hold the key to interventions which may regardless of whether slow down or alleviate age-related decay.

At the heart of the justification for pharmacologic approaches to longevity is an awareness that aging does not operate in homogenous manner among individuals. However, it is a process of changes that occur across a continuum ranging from the molecular to the systemic levels. Examples of such changes include genomic instability, telomere shortening, epigenetic changes, proteostasis loss, mitochondrial dysfunction, cellular senescence and deregulated nutrient sensing as some examples. Understanding these complex mechanisms helps to establish bases for the development of pharmacological approaches that would target specific molecular pathways implicated in the aging process.

Attempts to target these pathways with pharmacological interventions are looking at addressing the cause of age-related decline, rather than simply treating the symptoms of age-associated disease. Moreover, this proactive strategy is aimed not only at longevity extension but also healthy lifespan extension – the plural of years free from the constraints of chronic diseases and disability.

In pursuit of longevity, pharmacological treatment provides numerous benefits. First of all, they offer a systematic avenue of attacking several elements boiling down to the process of aging at the same time. For example, some compounds are a lover to pleiotropic effects and affect different cellular processes that are involved in aging and age-related diseases. Fourth, pharmacological interventions can be personalized into genetics as well as the environmental context of individuals; therefore, it could improve the effectiveness and safety. Moreover, they provide scalability and availability with the possibility of easy dissemination and implementation in various diverse communities.

Additionally, pharmacological interventions show some promise in modulating other approaches for enhanced lifespan and health span such as behavioral and nutrition interventions. These positive effects may become amplified when pharmacological intervention is applied as an adjunctive measure combined with metabolic health, physical activity, and dietary patterns interventions.

Nevertheless, pharmacological intervention in longevity must be taken carefully and with a high level of professionalism. Unexpected risk factors, unintended consequences, and ethical issues need to be closely scrutinized and mitigated. Additionally, the complicated nature of aging requires multidisciplinary cooperation and significantly advanced translational research approaches to close a gap between basic science findings at one end and clinical implementation at another.

the logic behind pharmacological interventions in longevity rests on deep insight into aging through the above process as a biological phenomenon that is modifiable. Targeted by specific pathways related to aging, these therapeutics may potentially broaden health span and lifespan with promising perspectives for improving the quality of life in an elderly population.

c) <u>Key Pathways and Targets</u>

While investigating the aging process and attempting to treat its sometimes-incurable effects, scientists identified a number of vital pathways and molecular targets that seem very promising for pharmacological approaches in longevity. These pathways, involved in cellular metabolism homeostasis, energy balance control, stress management and longevity become a very attractive target for novel pharmaceutics focused on making sure the longer lives of humans would be healthy.

Among these targets, the mTOR pathway can be considered the most outstanding. mTOR is a key controller of cell growth, metabolism, and protein production that integrates nutrient signals, growth factor signaling and signalosome activated by cell stress. Lifespan extension and healthy age-related decline have been ascribed to inhibition of mTOR activity in model organisms, justifying this pathway as a likely anti-aging target.

Another group of NAD+-dependent deacetylases, known as sirtuins, has also attracted much interest. Sirtuins, which function in different processes of the cells such as DNA repair and metabolism also act to extend lifespan among various model organisms. In preclinical studies, Sirtuins activators like resveratrol have been shown promise as anti-aging therapeutics.

The other important actor in the cellular energy balancing act and metabolic regulation is the AMP-activated protein kinase (AMPK). When activated, AMPK allows cells to become more resistant to the stress resulting from energy deprivation and increases the rate of ATP generation while inhibiting ATP-consuming processes. It provides evidence that pharmacological activation of AMPK increases lifespan and enhances metabolism in model systems, thus suggesting a possible avenue for anti-aging interventions.

The role of the insulin/IGF-1 signaling pathway is related to controlling metabolism, growth, and aging. Decreased activity through this pathway has been linked to prolonged lifespan and improved health span in model organisms, encouraging the use of interventions that target modifications of insulin/IGF-1 signaling as a potential avenue for antiaging strategies.

Autophagy, a process by which cells degrade and recycle various aged or defective cellular species to maintain homeostasis as being integral to the aging process. Increased autophagy by pharmacological approaches is associated with extra lifespan and health span in some model organisms.

The role of the mitochondria in cellular energy production and metabolism decreases with age to explain this process. Various approaches that can be used to maintain mitochondrial function or even boosts Mito Biogenesis are prospective anti-aging interventions.

The phenomenon of cellular senescence defined by irreversible cell cycle arrest and with a different spectrum of secretory phenotype plays an important role in making physiological changes associated with aging and age-related diseases. Specifically, elimination or SASP modulation through senolytic agents can increase longevity thus leading to healthy aging.

The unveiling of important pathways and targets that play critical roles in regulating aging has provided promising opportunities for the creation of pharmacological intervention products, which have potential to promote a healthy ageing phenomenon as well as increase longevity. In addition, investigation of these pathways and modulation of them may give opportunity to change the attitude towards aging as well as age-related diseases opening new perspective for future where elderly become not only inevitable but manageable.

d) Promising Pharmacological Agents

To achieve the goal of prolonging human lifespan and improving healthspan, the scientists have ventured into pharmacology by investigating several drugs that may show unique properties. This mission has resulted to the search of various important substances, each having distinct mechanisms and benefits. These include rapamycin, metformin, resveratrol, nicotinamide adenine dinucleotide (NAD +) precursors, senolytics and calorie restriction mimics. Decoding the mechanisms and consequences of these pharmacological agents is deemed essential in clarifying potential Utility for human well-being and longevity.

Rapamycin, a macrolide compound first discovered in soil samples collected on Easter Island and found to inhibit the mechanistic target of rapamycin (mTOR) signaling pathway, has received much attention. In this regard, rapamycin regulates cell functions that are associated with growth, metabolism promotes aging. This is also true to metformin a widely used medication for type 2 diabetes that has proven promising as an anti-aging agent because it activates AMPK (adenosine monophosphate-activated protein kinase), which is involved in the regulation of lifespan.

Resveratrol is a well-known polyphenolic compound and has been studied in terms of the benefits which have resulted from this supplement, mainly, its ability to activate Sirtuins which are proteins that help regulate cellular homeostasis and longevity. In addition, compounds that act as precursors of nicotinamide adenine dinucleotide (NAD+), such as nicotinamide ribosides and nicotinamide mononucleotides have been central in reducing function of mitochondria supported by cellular resistance.

Senolytics can be referred to as a new generation of drugs that are targeting senescent cells as they accumulate with time and lead to age-related pathologies. Senolytics with the ability to clear these dysfunctional cells has a tremendous potential in alleviating age-related deterioration and improving tissue regeneration. Moreover, calorie restriction mimetics like resveratrol and metformin mimic such calorie restriction dietary intervention as a way of extending lifespan in many organisms by modulating the metabolic pathways leading to cellular stress resistance.

Most of the research that has been done on such pharmacological agents have been based on the preclinical models, but with all that there is increasing interest in translating these findings into applied clinical applications for human health. Nevertheless, difficulties persist in the way of evaluating safety, efficacy and long-term consequences of these compounds applied to human beings. Strict clinical trials and interdisciplinary collaborations are needed to clarify the functionality of these pharmacological agents that promote health aging and increase human ageing in terms of years.

Age-related diseases are likely to see more action as pharmacological agents target diverse pathways in drug discovery with the objective of revolutionizing approaches and improving quality of life for all. Thus, researchers intended to untangle the complex mechanisms of aging and lifespan hoping that in the future people will be able not just to comprehend ageing but also manage it successfully or even turn back this process by means of pharmacological intervention.

e) Challenges and Considerations

The aim to extend human life through the use of pharmacological interventions brings a lot of challenges and considerations, thereby contributing to the evolution landscape for longevity research. Although the possible advantages are close at hand, unfortunately much attention and consideration must be utilized to navigate through the path offering effective and safe interventions.

Heightening the very peak of these challenges is the paramount safety issue. Employing pharmacological agents designed to promote longevity requires careful assessment accompanied by stringent testing with a view of avoiding unintended harm. The level of toxicity profiles, expected negative impacts and the possibility of the emergence of unintended results should be conducted in depth to preserve people's health.

The other key consideration is efficacy. In theory, interventions look promising but must justify their implementation based on concrete benefits in terms of longer lifespan. Reliable clinical trials and representative longitudinal studies are critical to determine the effectiveness of pharmacological interventions in various ethnic groups and in different age categories.

The dosage optimization becomes an essential aspect of dealing with the longevity pharmacology challenges. Finding the best dosage that will help achieve the greatest benefits with minimal side effects is a balancing act of sorts, and, by and large, it must be determined accurately. The formation of therapeutic windows and dose-response relationships is crucial to govern the clinical practice in an appropriate direction.

However, the possible side effects have a formidable presence in longevity pharmacology. Infusion of exogenous agents into the complex biochemical environment created by human beings possesses an inbuilt tendency to initiation of side effects. Can not underestimate the importance of vigilant monitoring and surveillance to promptly detect and treat adverse events.

Drug interactions present another problem, especially one involving older age cohorts that typically suffer from a wide range of comorbidities and polypharmacy. The possibility of pharmacokinetic and pharmacodynamics interactions points out the need for comprehensive medication reconciliation and personalized treatment regimens.

The impact of longevity interventions extends to long-term effects, which constitute an especially challenging area of consideration. Longitudinal studies and post-marketing surveillance are needed to project the long-term effects of continued pharmacological interventions over prolonged periods because they would define precise benefits, as well as potential dangers.

All areas of longevity study and treatment stand upon ethical principles. Questions related to the issue of equity of access, informed consent and where desperate measures should be prioritized remain unanswered and make a transparent ethical framework for decision making absolutely necessary.

Additionally, the nature of aging itself requires a comprehensive response that goes beyond reductionist perspectives. Combine drugs in a number of different pathways that are associated with aging have potential but involve significant complexities regarding the composition, dosage, and regulation.

Heterogeneity of ageing, therefore, highlights the need for personalized medicine approaches focused on different genetic profiles, lifestyles and health differences. Precision interventions can deliver the best of both worlds — high efficacy with minimal downsides and this emerging paradigm ushers in a new age of longevity pharmacology.

Although the quest for pharmacological interventions in longevity carries with it immeasurable potentials, a plethora of multidimensional challenges and considerations are both entailed and meticulously required that call for teamwork among professionals across different fields. However, rational (through empirical research), moral (through ethical deliberation) and creative (innovative) discussions can only uncover the subtle complexities of aging and thus allow us to fully utilize longevity pharmacology.

CHAPTER 3
LIFESTYLE PRACTICES FOR LONGEVITY

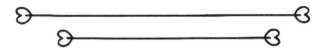

3.1.   Diet & Nutrition

D iet and nutrition define the integral corner that strengthens the quest for a better lifespan with day-to-day vigor and energy. As the last but not least, such intricate environment is a complex relationship including diet choices and physiological mechanisms to determine health outcomes, longevity and quality of life.

In this chapter, we discuss nutritional principles that would promote health and longevity in detail by focusing on diet patterns, foods rich in a given nutrient or best providing the whole required nutrients, as well as evidence-based approaches to optimally achieve desired efficiency.

- **<u>Understanding Dietary Patterns</u>**

Dietary patterns reflect on the entirety of foods and beverages that are consumed over time, which is a foundation of health and wellness. A person's choice of diet has a significant impact on health and life expectancy overall. Dietary pattern research attests to the importance of adopting diets rich in whole, nutrient-rich foods for maximum health benefits.

Of all the dietary patterns discussed, the Mediterranean is the epitome of health. It focuses on the intake of vegetative products such as fruit and vegetables, legumes, nuts and entire cereals. The addition of olive oil that provides monounsaturated fats is good for cardiovascular health. Consuming reasonable amounts of fish and poultry provide necessary proteins and omega-3 fatty acids, which ensures proper cognitive function and heart health. Alternatively, low intake of red meat and processed foods reduces the risk for chronic diseases associated with cardiovascular disease (CVD), type 2 diabetes, and certain types of cancers.

The health and longevity benefits derived from the Mediterranean diet are attributable to nutrients and phytonutrients. These bioactive components provide antioxidative, anti-inflammatory and metabolic control functions supporting body immune response against age-associated degeneration and pathological processes.

In addition, the Mediterranean lifestyle does not only involve food selection but also integrates other elements of physical activity, social networks and stress management. Various holistic health approaches emphasize the connectedness of certain lifestyle factors in promoting general wellness.

The comprehension of dietary patterns requires understanding the cultural, social and individual forces that shape eating habits. Fostering lifestyle habits associated with a diet diversified, harmonized and temperate, people can promote their health and longevity.

- **Key Nutrients for Health and Longevity**

Prevention of many ailments, maintenance of vitality and longevity all rely on the right nutrient uptake that is required for these functions as well as in prevention of life threatening complications. The range of the essential nutrients is made up from the micronutrients and macronutrients, which key to cell safety, metabolic stability and overall life quality.

The vitamins and minerals are micronutrient reservoirs, guiding by the hand vital biochemical processes needed for good health. Similarly, Vitamin D (also called the Sunlight vitamin) is involved in calcium absorption regulation bone health and plays a role in immune function. Vitamin D, the deficiency in which links to increased predisposition to autoimmune morbidities osteoporosis and certain cancers. Vitamin B12 which is essential for that the nervous system and supplies off hormones to maintain red blood cell production can only be found in animal-based foods with its origins being derived from animals fortified products. Vitamin B12 deficiency can be seen through fatigue, neurotropic disturbance and anemia.

Calcium is another essential mineral that increases bone strength and helps the muscle facilitate their function nerve send signals as well as signal the hormones. The lack of calcium is predisposing to increased risk in the development of osteoporosis and fractures-especially among aged populations.

Omega-3 fatty acids have a strong anti-inflammatory profile due to their long chain higher polyunsaturated eicosatetraenoic acid (EPA) and docosahexaenoic acid (DHA). This omega-3, protects from cardiovascular diseases. Omega-3 fatty acids are widely known as among the most abundantly available in fat tissues where they help to boost cardiovascular health, neurological processes and mood stabilization.

Focusing on nutrient-laden, vitamin/mineral rich, high quality proteins, complex carbohydrates, and healthy fats builds resiliency against age related degeneration of the vital body systems as well as mitigation of chronic diseases. The essence of having diverse nutrients sources is the utilization which in with eliminates all sorts of nutrition deficits that may lead to a wide range of complications for both young and old depending on their age.

- **<u>Strategies for Optimal Nutrition</u>**

In striving for an optimal diet, one is advised to practice awareness in what he or she eats, such as behavior that agrees with proof based nutritional standards. It is that upon strategizing, strategies ought to be based on the deliberate selection of foods that have spectra of important nutrients essential for maintaining health and vigour.

The key foundation of these approaches includes the use of a wide range of nutrient-rich foods in one's daily routine. Nutrient density consists in the rates of nutrients relative to the calorie level of a particular food. Through favoring food sources that are high in nutrition, people can increase their vitamin, mineral, antioxidant and other micro nutrient intake ensuring adequate amounts of the compounds required for optimal physiological functioning.

Unprocessed products govern the leading nutrition methods as opposed to refined and sweetened which most people prefer. Whole foods maintain their natural purity, having a cocktail of vitamins and fiber which are usually removed during feeding products. Notably, by choosing items such as the whole grains, fruits, vegetables, lean proteins and healthy fats individuals can not only increase their intake of nutrients but also lower chances to suffer from problems like the obesity diabetes and cardiovascular illness.

In addition, the evidence-based nutritional recommendations also guides as a guide to follow in terms of nutrient choices. These recommendations, based on scientific knowledge and expert judgments provide an essential system of evidence-based dietary guidelines for ideal nutrition. Keeping up to date and knowledgeable about such guidelines enable using the referred portion sizes, guide macronutrient distribution and obtain balance through diet.

Basically, this was the essence of optimal nutrition strategies to be inclusive of a total nutritional approach to food choice and eating patterns. With emphasis on nutrient density, whole foods and evidence-based practice the habit formation is geared toward health, longevity and achievement of vigor.

- **Plant-Based Nutrition**

Plant-based nutrition has turned out to be an attractive way of living that is known for its ability to improve one's health and freedom from illnesses associated with aging. The crux of plant-based diet is the fact that it focuses more on diets which are obtained from plants like vegetables, legumes and whole grains while reducing or avoiding animal foods.

There is a characteristic and significant benefit in plant-based nutrition due to its wealth of fiber, antioxidants, as well as the phytochemicals that are found in plants. Fiber aids digestive health, controls blood sugar levels and increases satiety – the feeling of fullness after meal – promoting weight control to combat against chronic disease like diabetes and heart disease.

Besides, antioxidants and phytochemicals that are readily available in high percentages of fruits, vegetables and other plant sources have profound anti-inflammatory effects as well as the ability to fight diseases. Determined by this the compounds aid in defeating oxidative tension, neutralizing free radicals and supporting body defenses against cardiovascular disease, cancer and other age associated conditions.

The adoption of an herbivore dietary pattern thereby will provide the necessary health and longer life spanning. Nevertheless, care needs to be taken that enough quantity of nutrients are consumed which is otherwise provided through animal products only like protein, iron, calcium and vitamin B12. Include plant-based sources of proteins, such as lentil, soybeans, tofu, tempeh and quinoa to ensure an adequate protein intake along with the fulfillment of other nutrient needs while providing the opportunity for dietary balance and diversity.

Plant-based nutrition provides an innovative perspective, motivated by a desire to improve health outcomes and prolong life. Through the adoption of healthful consumption habits with plant-based foods as preferred sources that contain fiber, antioxidants, and phytochemicals for a nourishing body healthy dietary pattern minimizing chronic disease risk while supporting sustainable wellbeing.

- ## **The Role of Phytonutrients**

Phytonutrients form a pillar in terms of nutrition and health, which runs into a broad variety of advantages beyond food's provision.

Phytonutrients are the plant compounds derived from the Greek word Phyto, which means plants and they include large numbers of bioactive substances present in fruits, vegetables, grains, nuts/seeds and herbs. They have several beneficial properties, the most outstanding of which are their antioxidative and anti-inflammatory effects, leading to the maintenance of cell integrity and combating ageing.

Pioneering phytonutrients effectiveness is flavonoids, carotenoids and polyphenols which each elements feature unique mechanism of action together with therapeutic implications. Containing more than 6000 bioactive products, flavonoids are a major constituent of berries, citrus fruits and leafy vegetables that play an antioxidant role by capturing radicals, thus protecting cells from oxidative damage associated with progenesis of chronic diseases and aging. It is carotenoids that give food its brilliant color and, apart from that, act as preforms of vitamin A necessary for vision development and one's general immunity. Polyphenols are present in tea, cocoa and spices and are known to reduce inflammation which alleviates systemic inflammation caused by chronic conditions such as cardiovascular disease as well as neurodegenerative diseases that cause cognitive impairment.

Body is fueled by a diverse palette of foods rich in phytonutrients, on which any healthy diet is crowned with multiple benefits to health and living. Moreover, phytonutrients are known for their antioxidant activity and ability to suppress inflammation. Studies have shown that phytonutrient intake can benefit the immune system, improve detoxification processes as well as lower the risk of chronic diseases such as cancer and diabetes. The adoption of a prone dietary pattern highlights the emphasis on culinary diversity and seasonal products, implying a reciprocity between human healthiness from the specific voice natural environment.

Phytonutrients epitomize the transformative power of plant-based nutrition, offering a potent arsenal against the ravages of time and disease. Through mindful dietary choices that prioritize colorful fruits, vegetables, and whole grains, individuals can harness the extraordinary potential of phytonutrients to thrive and flourish throughout the aging process.

- **Nutritional Considerations for Aging**

In the impact of time and its relentless flow onwards, bringing in the process of growing old with a range of physiological shifts that call for delicate controlling alterations so as to maintain vigor and health. At the juncture of this paradigm change, a number of essential issues regarding nutrient ingestion, metabolic processes, as well as musculoskeletal quality are in play and these come into focus to define for the nutritional profile of older people.

At the center of nutritional perimeter of aging, is the analysis that metabolic needs keep changing with advancing decades, so also digestive abilities that cease to function well at certain point in time and may fall far short while limiting absorption as well as utilization. Features which promote less gastric acid excretion, decreased taste perception and ineffective nutrient transport emphasizes the need for highly digestible nutrients with high amount of assimilation. As a result, dietary regimes focusing on leanness and high meat proteins, whole grains and vitamin-dense vegetables can counteract the effect of age-related losses in body muscle mass, bone density and metabolic efficacy.

Notably, when viewed as a major component in the therapeutic nutrition arsenal against sarcopenia—the insidious muscular atrophy associated with growing old – protein rises above others. With the inclusion of good protein foods like lean meat, fish, eggs legumes and dairy in every meal, aging people can build skeletal muscle to support their body as prevent them from functional decline thus saving mobility necessary for independence even while they are old.

In addition, dehydration and further electro impulse resulting from age-related suspension to thirst perception.

3.2.   Exercise and Physical Activity

Over life generations, exercise and physical activity remain crucial for maintaining health and fitness throughout the ages, but most crucially when one grows older. The range of benefits that physical activity brings to human health includes the improvement of cardiovascular functioning, promotion of mobility, as well as maintaining cognitive functions for longevity. In this sub-chapter, we discuss the significance of workout in age groups regarding an ability preserves your mobility, buoyancy and life quality.

- **The Importance of Exercise in Aging**

It becomes more and more evident to people while aging that doing exercises is crucial for a physical and mental state of being. Aging is usually characterized by a whole lot of physiological changes such as moderations in muscle mass, bone density and cardiovascular condition. Nevertheless, the importance of regular workout and physical activity in responding to this age-related decline has always been underscored by research.

Exercise represents one of the main pillars in maintaining independence and a good life among prisoners. Research findings point to the potential of structured exercise programs in reducing aging-related chronic diseases like cardiovascular disease, diabetes type 2, and osteoporosis. Elders who embark on physical activities can save themselves from the development and advancement of these immobilizing conditions thereby extending their life span by making them more vigorous.

Also, the exercise is accompanied by numerous physiological adaptations which are obviously advantageous for the subject of this age. These help to retain muscle strength and flexibility which are vital in continuing mobility while avoiding functional restrictions. Furthermore, exercise leads to better cardiovascular performance thus decreasing the chances of such diseases as they are associated with problems in this particular organ.

Secondly, the psychological advantages of physical activities are important to note as well. Physical activity has also been linked to relief from depression and anxiety, two mental health conditions common among senior individuals. Through feelings of accomplishment and wellbeing, exercise also helps in increasing the quality life satisfaction of ageing adults.

The role that exercise plays in old age cannot be emphasized enough. It is also a foundation of sustaining physical functionality, self-determination and complete wellness. With the regular participation in exercising and other physical activities, the older adult can even beat old age by enjoying a profound life into their golden years.

- ## **Enhancing Mobility and Functionality**

The maintenance of mobility and functional capacity assumes special importance in older adults as they provide the sense of independence and quality life. Impaired muscle strength, flexibility and balance associated with aging can substantially limit an individual's capability to carry out his or her daily activities compellingly in addition to navigating the environment safely.

In this respect, exercise appears as a potent asset that engenders improvements in mobility and functionality among the older generation. These elements that include strength training, flexibility exercises and balance drills play a major role in exercise programmes aimed at age-related declines in physical function. Particularly, strength training helps to keep the muscle mass and strength, which supports functional capacity and ADLs performance among older adult people.

Flexibility exercises ensure that the joint is well-maintained for its mobility and range of motion, thereby minimizing stiffness or discomfort arising from old age. In the process of engaging in exercise, seniors should include some stretching exercises to improve their flexibility and relieve such musculoskeletal limitations that can limit mobility.

In addition, balance drills play an important role in preventing falls as one of the major issues among geriatric group. Balance and proprioception exercises heighten the sense of stability and coordination level, which decreases falls' occurrence to minimize injuries.

Activity is a catalyst that provides improvement in mobility and functional ability among the aged individuals. In making declines in strength, flexibility and balance less of a problem for older people to rely on themselves as they engage in activities that are important to them and therefore managing their everyday lives with self-confidence. Older adults can enhance their functional performance and have a rewarding life even in their late years by continuing to take part in exercises suitable for them.

- **<u>Strength Training for Musculoskeletal Health</u>**

Strength training, better known as resistance training, is integral to maintaining musculoskeletal health now and especially later in our lives. However, this is a type of activity that involves following particular procedures aimed to stimulate different muscle groups with the use of weights, resistance bands or one's own body weight.

Besides, its importance is not only in increasing the muscular mass but even to strengthening the bones' density, it increases also physical strength and endurance.

Strength training offers great potential for the elderly to avert the inevitable decrease of muscle mass and bone tissue density, which is associated with aging. Therefore, people get old and it produces two problems related to their biology: sarcopenia (gradual decay of muscular tissue) as well as osteoporosis (weakened bones prone to fractures). The seniors can help to reduce such effects by incorporating resistance exercise training into their routines; thereby, preserving functional independence and decreasing the risk of falls and fractures.

Strength training has benefits beyond physical strength building. It motivates the sense of freedom and confidence, which enables individuals to perform their daily duties more conveniently and rapidly. Secondly, it assists in weight control, improves metabolism and cardiovascular performance. Not only can older adults improve their physical health via consistent strength training, but such regular exercise has the capacity to permanently transform a frailer and feebler mindset into one more resilient enough to welcome the trials of aging with enthusiasm and energy.

Essentially, strength training is the very essence of musculoskeletal health providing a wellspring to life depicted by longevity and resilience and ultimately tendering improved quality of living. Through the life-reviving force of resistance training, a person's body gains protective strength against old age and paves the way to a healthy lifestyle that thrives with time.

- **Flexibility and Range of Motion Exercises**

Flexibility and ROM exercises are an essential part of multiple fitness plans, especially those designed for persons who want to keep their musculoskeletal wellness as they advance in age. These movements work on flexibility of joints, muscles elasticity and general mobility to fight the natural tendency of stiffen of age (joint) and loss(muscles) over time.

When people grow old their chances of having a less motion range increase, affecting everyday life that can originate pain and lead to musculoskeletal discomfort or injury. Through implementing stretching exercises, doing yoga, tai chi and other flexibility-related activities in their daily routine, people can work against the process of aging on their musculoskeletal systems.

Most stretching exercises are aimed at specific parts of the body such that the muscle fibers become elongated and flexibility is increased. By practicing stretching on a regular basis, people can release muscle stiffness and ensure correct posture as well as better movement of the body in general. Yoga and tai chi, grounded in ancient practices, focusing on free-flowing movements and mindfulness of breath control to increase flexibility, create balance due and provide mental purity.

Furthermore, other advantages provided by flexibility and range of motion exercises are not directly connected with physical mobility. They have stress-relieving properties, facilitate relaxation and lead to clarity of thoughts and balance in the emotional state. Through mindfulness and awareness of the body, people learn to overcome what they face in the process of getting old with grace, but in high spirit.

- **<u>Balance and Stability Training</u>**

However, the need for balance and stability cannot be overemphasized among all individuals regardless of age especially as they get older to try to prevent falls or mobility issues. Balance training exercises have a powerful role in proprioception, coordination as well as postural control all of which greatly reduce the incidence of accidents and improve quality of life.

Age decreases the proprioception i.e., sense of position and movement, therefore balance training in older adults becomes necessary. Stability exercises, including one-limb standing, heel-toe walking, as well as balance boards intending proprioceptive feedback make people more aware of body actions and positions. Through such practices, seniors can better develop the reflex mechanism in reaction to sudden balance shifts and achieve stability under various conditions.

Balance training, which focuses on coordination as a necessary aspect of balance, develops through practice-based techniques that necessitate synchronization and efficient muscle activation. The physical exercises help not only to develop coordination but also inspire confidence regarding one's ability to walk around safely.

The ability to maintain a standing pose against gravity is called postural control, an essential function in maintaining balance and ensuring independence to prevent falling. The muscles that posture also include the core and lower body muscles which are strengthened through balance training exercises, reinforcing better alignment and stability.

Therefore, balance and stability training constitute one of the primary sources of fall avoidance approaches and contribute to maintaining mobility and independence among the elderly. These exercises can help people decrease their risk of falls, strengthen self-confidence, and maintain a higher quality of life long after they have reached the age retirement.

- ### Cardiovascular Exercise for Heart Health

Cardiovascular exercise or aerobic exercise is one of the foundational elements on proper heart health and human body's wellbeing. One can play different games such as walking cycling, swimming, and dancing which strengthen the muscle of heart hence improve circulation and regulation blood pressure lowers the risk of diseases in cardiovascular.

The heart's ability to pump blood into the body, nutrients which are carried by this blood is sustainably increased with regular cardiovascular exercise or aerobic training. The newfound ability, which translates to enhanced endurance and lower instances of fatigue during everyday activity, is a result of this increased efficiency.

Also, aerobic exercise can be said to aid in weight control since it entails the process of burning calories and enabling stored fat to be used up as energy. It also increases the production of endorphins, chemicals found inside your brain which are neurotransmitters that induce a sense of euphoria and relieves stress in order to promote positive feelings of well-being and concentration.

Not only do the cardiovascular exercises help with physical health, but the benefits include cognitive functioning. It was confirmed by researches that once a day aerobic exercise is of benefit for memory concentration and whole brain health mainly because it facilitates increased blood flow to the brain and promotes new neuron growth.

3.3. Stress Management Techniques: Mitigating the Effects of Chronic Stress on Health

Chronic stress has emerged as an integral element of modern society which impacts on people from every sector and sociodemographic group. Although stress is a normal and reflex reaction to external pressure, chronic exposure to avoidable stressors may have grave implications for health of an individual physically mentally as well as emotionally.

As this problem continues to be a growing concern, the answer emerged in the adoption of stress management techniques that is effective at managing chronic stress to maintain health and resilience.

- <u>Understanding Chronic Stress: A Modern Epidemic</u>

In the modern world, stress has evolved into a ubiquitous phenomenon that manifests in the form of persistent firing of the body's stress response system. In contrast to acute stress, which is a short-term reaction and often the product of an immediate threat, chronic stress results from consistent exposure to demanding conditions that span a diverse range of aspects in life, such as workload, financial pressure, family conflict and personal health. It seeps into the everyday reality, becoming an admixture of the human life and influencing people's health really much.

The great feature of chronic stress is that the period of time when it continues significantly exceeds the required duration to overcome generating factors. It works in the manner of a silent attacker, gradually sapping physiological resilience and psychological harmony. People caught up in its loop usually find themselves stuck in a vicious cycle of tension and pressure, with no relief point from the pressures around their circumstances.

Chronic stress throws out of gear the delicate equilibrium between the various mechanisms involved in responding and adapting to stressful stimuli, thereby perpetuating hyperarousal and hypersensitivity. The chronic activation of stress hormones, such as cortisol and adrenaline, further aggravates a state of hyperarousal where the body reacts physically more vigorously to threats. Sustained activation leads to dysfunctions of many organ systems, disrupting their normal functioning and damaging the health balance.

The omnipresence of chronic stress highlights its relevance as a contemporary pandemic, therefore demanding holistic understandings regarding it varies mechanisms and implications. Combating chronic stress calls for a holistic approach: individuals need to find ways of adapting while the society itself should seek opportunities through which it can relieve some of these overarching pressures—those that define modern day life. Through undoing the layers of chronic stress, we can create an opportunity for a better and more enhanced life in the future.

- ## The Impact of Chronic Stress on Health

The negative impacts of chronic stress on health result in sweeping throughout all areas of wellness. The key component in this process is the imbalance of stress hormones such as cortisol and adrenaline, which conducts the body reflexive reaction to long-term hardship.

The chronic elevation of the level of cortisol affects this delicate system equilibrium and, thereby predisposing people to infections as well as diseases. Additionally, non-resolving stress leads to inflammation which has been shown in chronic conditions including cardiovascular disease and metabolic disorders.

Chronic stress has to load the cardiovascular system, as high levels of cortisol are involved in increases of blood pressure and heart rate that makes these individuals more vulnerable to hypertension, atherosclerosis and coronary diseases. Physiologically, chronic stress promotes insulin resistance and impairs glucose metabolism, hence the predisposition to diabetes and obesity.

In addition, long periods of stress are deleterious to mental wellbeing as they lay the grounds for anxiety disorders and depression among other psychiatric conditions. The continuous stream of stressors undermines emotional resilience, triggering a sequence of negative feelings and rational misconceptions.

Chronic stress affects the body in various ways and complicates every aspect of physiological and psychological health. Conquering this ubiquitous threat requires a comprehensive framework, including both personal stress-management tactics and widespread societal efforts designed to create healthy conditions of life.

Through acknowledging the massive consequences of chronic stress, we can develop a world that values wellness and vitality in an ever-growing environment.

- **Effective Stress Management Techniques: Empowering Resilience and Well-being**

Stress levels continue to grow, and given this situation resilience development as well as the implementation of pro-active stress management techniques are crucial directions important for protection and promotion of health.

1. Mindfulness Meditation and Relaxation Techniques

Mindfulness meditation is based on ancient contemplative precepts whereby one would learn to pay attention to the present-moment awareness and is a giving act of accepting thoughts, feelings, physiological reactions objectively. Through the promotion of inner peace and tranquility, SMC practices can reduce physiological arousal generated by perceived stressors promoting emotional measures and resilience.

2. Cognitive-Behavioral Therapy (CBT)

CBT is a specific kind of structured, empirically supported psychotherapeutic intervention that targets changing the adaptive thinking and behaviors that perpetuates stress and emotional distress. CBT helps people to establish and develop self-efficacy through cognitive restructuring, behavioral activation, and skill-building techniques that enable them to cope with stressors by changing negative thoughts into productive responses.

3. Physical Activity and Exercise

Besides the physiological benefits that include obviation of such morbidities as hypertension, diabetes, cardiovascular diseases among others that individuals are bound to acquire with regularly exercises and physical activity assists in tackling one's stress as well. The muscular tension is reduced, the cortisol levels dropped and an increase of endorphin release (nature's natural medication for mood) and overall resistance to stress after aerobic exercise or strength training, yoga or tai chi.

4. Social Support and Connection

The establishment and maintenance of socially dependent network systems as well as meaningful interpersonal associations are crucial for protecting against the negative impacts that chronic stress unleashes. Spending good times with family and friends, counseling for emotional support, joining groups or support groups can promote sense of attachment, affirmation and community cohesion that stimulates positive psychological state as well as cause hardness.

5. Lifestyle Modifications and Self-Care Practices

By making healthy habits and self-care, human body strength will be fortified with its natural healing mechanism responding to chronic stressors. Some of the major aspects of helpful stress management and healthy self-care include sleeping enough, eating a well-balanced diet without adopting diets full with empty calories, practicing calming methods such as deep breathing or progressive muscle relaxation every day and setting realistic goals and limits.

The high level of chronic stress shows the need to start prophylactic management along with having a chance to protect health, bolster resilience, and raise well-being. Integrating mindfulness, cognitive-behavioral strategies, physical activity, social support and self-care practices within daily living resources individuals the ability to meet with equanimity and vitality of that which life brings.

As we pursue a comprehensive strategy of stress management, we can formulate a culture of wellness and resilience where chronic stress cannot prevail on us as individuals but live free lifestyles which are balanced, vital, and thriving.

3.4. Importance of Quality Sleep for Overall Well-Being and Longevity

With the buzz of our modern world, we often forget that good sleep is equally important. However, sleep is the cornerstone of health and vitality, contributing tremendously to physical and mental life. This section is devoted to the diverse value of sleep quality, its modifying influence on general state and length of life, and daily practice.

- ### The Foundations of Quality Sleep

The right quality of sleep is the foundation for human health; it goes far beyond those hours we spend in bed to include details about soundness, periods and when restorative cycles occur. In essence, the mechanism of quality sleep centers on the delicate orchestration between non-rapid eye movement (NREM) and rapid eye movements REM), which anchors varied respectively to repair processing restoration in cognition

The NREM sleep, being the early stages of function united with circadian cycle is an integral phase in which body performs numerous operations important to allow physical restoration and upkeep. Such stage helps in tissue healing, muscle regeneration and immunoregulation. It acts as a significant stage for the body to heal from all wear and tear that has been accrued during the day, with complete physiological functioning attained following awakening.

On the other hand, REM sleep takes place during late stages of a sleeping cycle and it is mostly considered in connection with processes that concern cognitive functions, consolidation as well as emotional regulation. Information that is collected during the whole day, goes through the processing of being refined memories and work on learning processes can only take place during REM sleep. Furthermore, REM sleep helps in rebalancing the moods and emotional state of an individual contributing to mental resilience.

The different stages in sleep represent a delicate balance that needs to be attained through disrupted working faster leads to impairment on the capacities of cognitive, emotional and physical one. The understanding of the continuum and its maintenance through routine sleep hygiene habits which include regularity in sleeping time, establishing a supportive environment for sound slumber as well as minimizing excitants just before one dozes will help maximize quality deep rest key to healthy being.

- **Physical Health Benefits of Quality Sleep**

Notably, sleep deprivation or poor-quality sleep have been linked to an increased risk of developing hypertension, heart disease, obesity and type 2 diabetes among other long term health conditions. Sleep is a critical period for the body in which it regulates hormone levels such as appetite and metabolism. Failing to maintain such a balance can contribute to weight gain and even insulin resistance leading to metabolic dysfunction resulting into a good environment for metabolic disorders' development.

Additionally, chronic sleep loss results in immune system impairment that reduces resistance to pathogens (pathogen) and undermines the body's ability mount an effective immune response. In individuals experiencing chronic sleep deficits, such susceptibility to infections and illness increases significantly revealing that sound sleeping patterns are fundamental in boosting the body's innate defense mechanisms.

Moreover, constant sleep deprivation has an impact on the immune system by making it difficult for the body to fight off diseases and produce a functional immune system. The heightened susceptibility to infectious illnesses is more evident in people with persistent sleep deficits. This highlights the importance of having enough sleep-in order to strengthen the innate immunity of our bodies.

Finally, with regard to wholistic health and well-being, one such element would be putting first and securing ones' slumber's quality as it directly affects physical endurance capacity, mental alertness state and psychological steadiness. People can therefore strive towards living better lives by incorporating restorative sleep habits into their daily routines, while appreciating that such sleeps play a critical role in maintaining optimal physiological function for improved vitality and longevity.

- **<u>Cognitive Function and Emotional Well-being</u>**

Some other facts that support the need for quality sleep are not only that it is an effective tool in maintaining a healthy body but also plays a huge role in how we think and feel. In order to protect mental health, sleep is a complex process that changes as the mind goes through various stages of sleep.

In different phases of sleep, brain processes and consolidates the information got during the day hence promoting memory retention as well as learning. Memory consolidation is important for encoding memories and extracting core data that improves subsequent cognitive performances. Sufficient slumber is necessary so that the brain can store details well and recall them when needed; thus, attention span increases.

Sleep also has a strong connection with emotional balance. It regulates emotional responses enabling individuals manage stress, anxiety and mood swings efficiently. Sleep deprivation upsets this equilibrium causing increased emotional reactivity, irritability and inability to cope with regular stressors. The ability of our brains to keep our emotions under control therefore gets compromised making us less judgmental towards others and more prone to interpersonal difficulties.

The quality sleep fosters cognitive resilience and emotional well-being by allowing the brain to function optimally. It provides the necessary foundation for mental clarity, emotional stability, and overall psychological health. Therefore, prioritizing adequate sleep is paramount for maintaining cognitive sharpness and emotional equilibrium in daily life.

- **Longevity and Quality of Life**

The correlation between sleep and longevity has garnered significant attention in longevity research, with compelling evidence highlighting its profound impact on overall health and well-being. Consistent, high-quality sleep is not merely a luxury but a fundamental determinant of longevity and vitality.

Studies consistently demonstrate that individuals who prioritize sufficient, restorative sleep tend to live longer and enjoy a higher quality of life compared to those with poor sleep habits. Quality sleep is associated with a myriad of health benefits, including reduced risk of chronic diseases such as cardiovascular ailments, diabetes, and obesity. Additionally, it enhances metabolic health, bolsters immune function, and promotes physical resilience against illnesses.

Moreover, quality sleep fosters mental acuity and emotional stability, enabling individuals to navigate life's challenges with clarity and composure. It replenishes cognitive resources, enhances problem-solving skills, and fosters creativity, contributing to a more fulfilling and productive life.

In conclusion, investing in quality sleep is not only a key component of longevity but also integral to enhancing the overall quality of life. By prioritizing sleep hygiene and establishing healthy sleep habits, individuals can unlock the full potential of longevity and enjoy a vibrant, fulfilling existence for years to come.

- **<u>Strategies for Enhancing Sleep Quality</u>**

In our fast-paced world, prioritizing quality sleep has become increasingly important for maintaining overall well-being and longevity. Adopting healthy sleep habits and implementing effective strategies can significantly improve sleep quality and promote optimal health outcomes.

1. Maintain a Consistent Sleep Schedule:

Establishing a regular sleep-wake cycle helps regulate the body's internal clock, promoting better sleep quality. Aim to go to bed and wake up at the same time every day, even on weekends, to reinforce your body's natural sleep rhythm.

2. Create a Relaxing Bedtime Routine:

Engage in calming activities before bedtime to signal to your body that it's time to wind down. This could include reading a book, taking a warm bath, or practicing relaxation techniques like gentle stretching or listening to soothing music.

3. Optimize Sleep Environment Conditions:

Create an optimal sleep environment by controlling factors such as light, temperature, and noise level. Keep your bedroom dark, cool, and quiet to facilitate uninterrupted sleep. Consider using blackout curtains, white noise machines, or earplugs if necessary.

4. Limit Exposure to Stimulating Activities Before Bed:

Avoid engaging in stimulating activities such as using electronic devices, watching TV, or working right before bedtime. The blue light emitted by screens can disrupt the body's natural sleep-wake cycle, making it harder to fall asleep.

5. Practice Stress Management Techniques:

Incorporate stress-reduction techniques into your daily routine to promote relaxation and ease into sleep. Techniques such as mindfulness meditation, deep breathing exercises, and progressive muscle relaxation can help calm the mind and body, making it easier to transition into restful sleep.

6. Monitor Dietary Habits:

Be mindful of your dietary choices, especially in the hours leading up to bedtime. Avoid consuming heavy meals, caffeine, or alcohol close to bedtime, as these substances can interfere with sleep quality and disrupt the sleep cycle.

CHAPTER 4
EXPLORING RAPAMYCIN

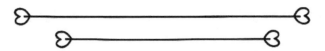

4.1. Origin and History of Rapamycin as an Immunosuppressant

In pharmacology, the most prominent is rapamycin which is also known as sirolimus. The history of its identity as an immunosuppressant agent uncovers a story of accidental discovery, careful analysis, and revolutionary therapeutic employment. Here, the beginning, formation and growth of Rapamycin as a major immunosuppressive drug is discussed following from a natural product to treatment leading breakthrough.

- **Discovery:**

The background of this discovery is the era of 1970s, and unfolds in the rough land full of uncommon biodiversity, that was Easter Island or Rapa Nui. Before this discovery, it was in the samples of soil from this isolated area that scientists noted a strange microorganism Streptomyces hygroscopicus. The secret to unleashing novel therapeutic possibilities existed, one that was held by these soil-residing bacteria, known for their capacity to release a wide variety of secondary metabolites.

Scientists at Ayerst Research Laboratories (now Wyeth Pharmaceuticals) in Canada began a journey to isolate Rapamycin upon realizing the pharmacological importance of Streptomyces hygroscopicus. Under the strict scrutiny of advanced experimentation and fermentation techniques, scientists managed to separate Rapamycin from the broth of this mysterious bacillus. This seminal finding marked the beginning of a new day in pharmacology as it opened up revolutionary strides in immunosuppression therapies.

- Immunosuppressive Properties:

After initially being heralded for its strong antifungal capabilities, Rapamycin soon garnered attention as an appealing prospect in the arena of immunosuppressive therapy. Its immunomodulatory effects were clarified because of the persistent scientific activity and critical analysis. In laboratory settings across the world, Rapamycin was shown by research to be the only agent having a unique disrupting effect on the activation and proliferation of Tlymphocytes, which are key components in the adaptive immune system.

Unlike classical immunosuppressants such as cyclosporine acting on upstream signalling events, Rapamycin stood out by engaging its action in the pathway beyond interleukin-2 (IL-2) signalling. Rapamycin targeted the mammalian target of rapamycin (mTOR) pathway selectively and was therefore a novel small molecule that offered great therapeutic potential in preventing rejection of organs following transplantation as well as managing autoimmune diseases.

Rapamycin's journey from the shores of Easter Island to the forefront of immunosuppressive therapy epitomizes the transformative power of scientific discovery and underscores the profound impact of natural products in shaping modern medicine.

- ## Clinical Development of Rapamycin

From preclinical studies demonstrating promise, rapamycin was part of a lineage which nurtured a hope that would reach transplant medicine. Its success story to go from lab biochemistry to a clinical indication reflects the painstaking process of clinical development.

Improving preclinical findings, clinical trials were conducted to determine the safety and efficacy of Rapamycin as a means of inhibiting organ rejection in transplant patients. These trials, characterized by precise planning and implementation aimed at illuminating Rapamycin's therapeutic potential in such a way to guarantee patient care.

The climax of these activities was in the year 1999 when U. A drug regulatory authority, namely Food and Drug administration or FDA approved the use of Rapamycin in renal transplantation which signified a metamorphosis in transplant therapeutics.

FDA's approval provided an important step, confirming the drug efficacy and safety profiles in a clinical environment. Over time, the therapeutic domain of Rapamycin was extended from renal transplants to liver and heart transplants, further strengthening its status as a pillar of transplant pharmacotherapy.

The clinical development of rapamycin highlights an integrated effort of researchers, clinicians and regulatory agencies. It highlights the importance of clinical trials in the ability to translate scientific advancements into real clinical benefits, rekindling hope once again to transplant recipients worldwide.

- <u>Mechanism of Action of Rapamycin</u>

The core of Rapamycin's immunosuppressive abilities lies in the pathway mechanism, interfering with the target of mammalian Rapamycin (m TOR). Chemically, Rapamycin forms a complex with FK-binding protein 12 (FKBP12), which binds and inhibits mTORC1 that regulates cell growth, proliferation and metabolism.

The mTOR pathway regulates cellular reactions to environmental stimuli and is thus mostly referred to as a signal integrator that dictates critical cell functions. As Rapamycin inhibits mTOR, it causes significant levels of immunosuppression modifying the immune system's attack on transplanted organs. This selective inhibition cuts down rejection reactions through minimizing systemic toxicity, one of the main characteristic assets of Rapamycin's therapeutic profile.

The specificity with which rapamycin targets mTOR promotes the idea that it could be a transplant medicine's core pillar. Its mechanism of action is a perfect example of the sophisticated balance between molecular pathways and therapeutic effects, exemplifying immunosuppressive pharmacology intricacy. Thus, the molecular scheme of action of rapamycin reveals a world filled with complexities that reveal pathways to innovation in therapies and medical care for transplantation.

- **Clinical Applications of Rapamycin**

Rapamycin, initially promoted for its strong immunosuppressive attributes in organ transplantation has moved an excessive way from traditional applications to become a potential therapeutic lead across many clinical spheres. Autoimmune diseases, such as rheumatoid arthritis and SLE, are one of the most important fields where Rapamycin effectively works: These two conditions are characterized by uncontrolled immunity hence difficult to treat. Rapamycin's selective suppression of the malignant immune reaction without undermining immunity as a whole is conditionally invaluable for disabling autoimmune-associated inflammation and tissue destruction.

This is in relation to autoimmune diseases whereby Rapamycin works through targeting the mechanistic target of rapamycin (mTOR) pathway which acts as a modulator for cellular functions like proliferation, metabolism and autophagy among others. As a result of effecting mTOR signaling, Rapamycin suppresses the overactivation of immune cells, hence reducing cytokine protein production and disease intensity. Its selective response of action is therapeutically favorable, leading to minimal adverse effects as compared to conventional immunosuppressive agents.

In addition, apart from its immunomodulatory effects, Rapamycin has various pharmacological properties that further enhance the range of its application. More and more evidence confirm its power in the fight against various malignancies, neurodegenerative diseases, and age-related conditions. The mTOR pathway, closely associated with cellular senescence and aging processes is functionally linked to rapid life-extension studies of Rapamycin. Rapamycin is an agent that may prevent mTOR-induced cellular senescence and increases autophagic activity, thus restoring age-related pathologies and contributing to longevity.

The clinical uses of rapamycin far surpass straightforward immunosuppression, comprising a broad armamentarium of autoimmune conditions and spreading to several therapeutic domains. Its selective modulation of the mTOR pathway not only supports its immunomodulatory effects but also highlights it as a candidate for cancer treatments, neurodegenerative and elderly-based conditions.

Looking forward, as researchers move deeper to understand its complexity, Rapamycin promises to remain a pillar in the emerging paradigm of precision medicine and therapeutic advancement.

4.2. Understanding the Mechanism of Action: Inhibition of the mTOR Pathway

The mechanistic target of rapamycin (mTOR) pathway acts as a central regulator for cell growth, metabolism and proliferation. It acts as a signaling pathways which integrate multiple environmental cues, such as nutrient abundance, energy metabolism and growth signals to coordinate cellular response in order to preserve homeostatic conditions. mTOR is, therefore, a key modulator of fundamental cellular processes such as protein synthesis, autophagy, lipid metabolism and mitochondrial activity which make it to be an important regulatory determinant of fate and nature.

- Cell Growth and Metabolism of mTOR Signal.

The mTOR or the mechanistic target of rapamycin signaling regulates crucial cellular processes, especially in controlling growth and metabolism. Central to this signaling pathway is the mTOR protein kinase, which operates within two distinct complexes: For instance, mTOR Complex 1(mTORC1) and mTOR Complex 2 (mI-PRGDF). Included are mTORC1 that plays a crucial role in regulating cell growth and metabolic functions.

The activation of mTORC1 is a complex process that is driven by various stimuli including growth factors, for instance, insulin and insulin-like growth factor 1 protein along with other essential amino acids arid cellular energy level such as the ATP/AMP ratio. Then mTORC1 responds to these sensory cues by its activation and subsequent phosphorylation of downstream effectors such as S6K and 4E-BP1. This phosphorylation cascade leads to protein synthesis, which in turn stimulates cell division and accumulation.

In addition, mTORC1 coordinates numerous cues from the environment to regulate cellular metabolic reprogramming. Through control of protein synthesis, mTORC1 dictates the presence of metabolic enzymes as well as nutrient transporters that regulate conversion and uptake of nutrients in the cell.

In the dysregulation of mTOR signaling in many pathological conditions such as cancer, metabolic disorders, and neurodegenerative diseases. The knowledge of the complex workings mechanisms that underlie mTOR signalling opens up immense therapeutic avenues for these conditions.

- **Role of Rapamycin in Inhibiting mTOR Pathway**

The mTOR pathway has a potent inhibitor, namely Rapamycin that is a natural macrolide compound extracted from Streptomyces hygroscopicus. Its mechanism of action is very specific targeting mTORC1. This complex, known as rapamycin-FKBP12 is formed through the association of rapamycin with an intracellular protein called FK506-binding protein 12 (FKBP12).

This quaternary complex attaches to mTORC1 and transcribes its catalytic activity by allostery. Disruption of mTORC1 signaling mediated by rapamycin is a hindrance to downstream activities governed by the protein that include such processes as protein synthesis, cell growth and metabolic regulation.

The therapeutic value of rapamycin and the related drugs goes beyond their immunosuppressor functions. They show potential in treating several diseases that are marked with mis regulated mTOR signaling, namely some types of cancer, metabolic abnormalities and autoimmune disorders.

Nevertheless, one should keep in mind that the clinical applicability of rapamycin is dampened by its side effects and partial ability to work in some scenarios. Targeted therapies, especially based on rapamycin and inhibiting mTOR activities are currently being studied in ways that will help them to enhance their effectiveness in treating diseases related to mTOR.

- <u>**Effects of mTOR Inhibition on Cell Metabolism**</u>

The inhibition of mTOR (mechanistic target of rapamycin) by rapamycin has emerged as a pivotal intervention in understanding cellular metabolism. mTOR, a serine/threonine kinase, orchestrates various cellular processes, including protein synthesis, metabolism, and autophagy. Rapamycin, a potent mTOR inhibitor, induces profound alterations in cell metabolism, offering insights into fundamental cellular mechanisms.

At the heart of mTOR inhibition lies the suppression of protein synthesis, a hallmark effect mediated by rapamycin. mTORC1 (mTOR complex 1), a key downstream effector of mTOR, regulates protein synthesis through phosphorylation of its substrates, including S6K and 4E-BP1. Rapamycin effectively inhibits mTORC1, thereby curtailing the translational machinery responsible for synthesizing proteins crucial for cell growth and division. This attenuation of anabolic processes impedes cellular proliferation, offering a potential avenue for therapeutic intervention in conditions characterized by excessive cell growth, such as cancer.

Moreover, mTOR inhibition by rapamycin triggers autophagy, a dynamic cellular process essential for maintaining cellular homeostasis and integrity. Autophagy serves as a quality control mechanism, facilitating the degradation and recycling of damaged or dysfunctional cellular components. By enhancing autophagic flux, rapamycin promotes the clearance of damaged mitochondria and protein aggregates, mitigating cellular stress and bolstering cellular resilience. This mechanism underscores the role of rapamycin in mitigating age-related decline and promoting longevity by preserving cellular integrity and function.

- **Implications for Aging and Age-Related Diseases**

Rapamycin modulation of the mTOR pathway creates enormous scope in the development of therapeutical intervention for aging and age- related chronic disorders. Exchangeable discoveries among different model organisms have demonstrated the outstanding effects of rapamycin-induced mTOR suppression in lengthening lifespan and mitigating age-associated diseases. As a result, the activity of mTORC1 is suppressed by rapamycin, unleashing an array of downstream effects consistent with enhanced longevity and improved healthspan.

It addition, rapamycin has promising therapeutic applicability in the treatment of age diseases which include cancer, neurodegenerative disorder, cardiovascular and metabolic syndromes. By attacking the complicated molecular pathways involved in aging and disease pathogenesis rapamycin brings us a multifaceted form of intervention and rejuvenation. Notably, the capacity of rapamycin to regulate essential cellular functions such as protein synthesis, metabolism activity and autophagy establishes it is a valuable drug that has great applications in human health and longevity.

The inhibition of mTOR by Rapamycin heralds a new dimension in to understanding cellular metabolism and its implications on aging biology. Its diverse impact on cell metabolism as well as its correlation with aging and age-related syndrome underscores the potential therapeutic value of targeting mTOR pathways in counteracting physical delimitation associated with aging, and promoting healthy aging.

Rapamycin inhibits the mTOR pathway, which reflects a new concept in drug development by modulating cellular metabolism to increase life span. Rapamycin performs pleiotropic functions on cellular processes, including protein synthesis, autophagy and metabolism by damping mTORC1 signaling. Understanding the operation of these mechanisms, has significant meaning to our understanding about aging and age-related diseases presenting new window in terms of treatment strategies aimed at improving the healthspan as well vitality.

4.3. Mimicking Caloric Restriction: Implications for Lifespan and Health Span

The study likewise talks about the limitation of nutrient and its role in life-prolonging techniques. Caloric restriction is defined as a feeding regimen that reduces caloric intake while avoiding malnutrition, which has been shown to be associated with increased lifespan and reduced age-dependent disease in yeast through mammals. Although maintaining rigid caloric restriction regimens is often a demanding enterprise for many, researchers have looked to identify pharmaceutical interventions and lifestyle adaptations that mimic the effects of caloric restriction thereby identifying methods that offer enhanced lifespan and health span without strict necessity for drastic dietary restrictions.

- ### Understanding Caloric Restriction: A Foundation for Longevity Research

Caloric restriction, which should not lead to malnourishment, has been the focus of a particular interest among the researchers eager to unlock secrets of aging and longevity. Its massive implications for life extension, early-age disease prevention, and anti-aging have inspired vast scientific research that has worked to uncover the complex metabolic pathways involved in cellular senescence.

One of the critical features of caloric restriction is its inability to cause a metabolic switch within cells. Confronted with low energy supply, organisms have to opt for a number of adaptive mechanisms that promote cell survival and retain cellular homeostasis. A salient part of this metabolic adaptation entails the activation of stress response pathways specifically, including but not limited to AMP-activated protein kinase (AMPK) pathway that detects changes in cellular energy levels and coordinates appropriate responses for conserving energy and promoting cell resilience.

AMPK regulation initiates a series of steps designed to improve resistance to cellular stress conditions and extend longevity. This entails the induction of antioxidant defenses to counter oxidative stress, alongside autophagy activation – a sort of recycling process in cell organelles and protein aggregates. Further, by eliminating defective pieces of equipment, cells remain functional and fend off undesirable effects of aging.

In addition, caloric restriction activates the DNA repair pathways that causes proper genome maintenance and minimizes mutations which cause cancer due to aging. Improved DNA repair competence facilitates the adaptation of cells to endogenous and exogenous stress which may cause DNA damage, ensuring genome integrity and encouraging longevity.

The cell's powerhouse named mitochondria also play a central role in reducing the effects of caloric restriction on longevity. The mitochondrial function reduces with age, hence resulting in a steep increase in ROS and impaired energy production. Caloric restriction has been proven in some studies to improve mitochondrial biogenesis, increase the oxidative efficiency of mitochondria, and reduce oxidative stress while supporting cellular energy metabolism. This enhanced mitochondrial activity contributes to the general cellular wellbeing and makes cells more resistant to aging.

Moreover, apart from its impact on cellular metabolism and stress responses, caloric restriction affects systemic physiology to a profound degree since it notably alters various metabolic pathways and hormone signalling cascades. Caloric restriction has been demonstrated to enhance insulin sensitivity and decrease the levels of IGF-1; a hormone associated with healthy aging. Through that modulation of the biochemical pathways, caloric restriction can promote metabolic health and reduce disease risk to disorders such as diabetes and cardiovascular disease.

It has been associated with changes in nutrient-sensing pathways, such as the mTOR pathway – a mechanism that controls cell growth and proliferation by responding to availability of nutrients. Inhibition of mTOR signaling using caloric restriction delay the aging cellular process and induce longevity through preservation of cellular resources and re-routing energy towards maintenance and repair pathways.

The longstanding effects of caloric restriction on cellular metabolism, stress responses, and systemic physiology contribute to a favorable environment for longevity and healthy aging. Although the exact mechanisms underlying the effects of caloric restriction are still being investigated, its potential uses in health promoting universality and longevity are becoming more apparent.

- **Pharmacological Mimetics of Caloric Restriction: Unlocking the Potential of Rapamycin and Beyond**

Caloric restriction is an ancient practice still being praised for its influential capacity regarding health and longevity. However, its rigid diet demands make it inconvenient for most people. In addressing this threat, the field of pharmacology is aimed at discovering substances that can mimic calorie restriction phenomenon. Within this pool of agents, however, rapamycin stands out as a frontrunner with the capacity to transform longevity research and therapeutic interventions.

Although initially developed as an immunosuppressant, rapamycin's path from transplant medicine to the leading antiaging drugs reflects its inherent complexity. Fundamentally, it includes the suppression of mTOR pathway – a crucial onward directing cellular development, digestion, and maturing techniques. Through blocking mTOR signaling, rapamycin creates a metabolome in line with caloric restriction and this sets off a series of cascading molecular processes that result in a long life span as well as increased length of the health span.

One of the essential features of rapamycin's potency lies in its ability to reposition cellular metabolism towards a frugal, caloric-restriction-like state. By blocking the mTOR signaling pathway, rapamycin decreases anabolism and stimulates catabolism encouraging cells to focus on maintaining and repairing tissues rather than growing and multiplying. This metabolic transition, however, not only postpones age-related diseases but also provides resilience against numerous stressors that preserve organisms from the tyranny of time.

In addition, rapamycin's effect extends beyond the cellular borders and affects complex signal equation regulating systemic physiology. Ticking the key tissues of liver, adipose tissue, and brain with modulations of mTOR activity rapamycin makes a symphony of metabolic adaptations that collectively promote organismal health and longevity. Interestingly, the effect of rapamycin on autophagy—an integral proteomic process for cellular quality management—sheds light on the mechanistic connection between its molecular actions and anti-aging properties.

But the trials of rapamycin to be used in clinical translation are encumbered by a number of obstacles, primarily adverse effect and dose-dependent toxicity. The fact that rapamycin possesses immunosuppressive qualities, which have proven incredibly useful in transplant medicine, is indicative of widespread concern regarding susceptibility to infections and impaired wound healing when employed on a chronic basis. More, the dichotomous nature of mTOR signaling – that it exerts both pro and anti-aging actions – margins therapeutic scope by necessi-tati-ng precise modulation M nitrogen activity to hold its advantages while avoiding its defects.

With rapamycin, a number of pharmacological agents have been shown to serve as potential mimetics of caloric restriction representing distinctly individualized pharmacodynamic profiles and therapeutic prospects. Metformin is a key stand among various therapies available for combating type 2 diabetes and has received attention for activating AMPK, an enzyme that regulates cellular energetics.

By repeating some of the essential metabolic effects of calorie restriction, it is possible to formulate with metformin as a multifaceted application against age-related pathology but has its other boundaries and warnings.

In the same vein, resveratrol is an attracter of attention among scientists as this polyphenolic compound found in red wine has been claimed to promote sirtuin enzymes which are known mediators for caloric restriction's benefits. The clinical use of resveratrol is marred by controversy despite its pleiotropic effects on metabolism and aging; however, it faces challenges such as bioavailability and translation difference between preclinical models and human trials.

On the path for pharmacological mimickers of caloric restriction, it is inevitable to take this road with caution cognizant enough of the intricacies in molecular biology and therapeutic intervention. However, rapamycin and its analogs have amazing potential as age-promoting intervention tools; however, their usage requires a more complex understanding of action mechanisms safety features and interactions with established treatment protocols.

The pursuit of longevity-enhancing interventions continues unabated, fueled by the collective ambition to defy the inexorable march of time. Through the convergence of pharmacology, molecular biology, and translational medicine, the quest for pharmacological mimetics of caloric restriction heralds a new era in the pursuit of ageless vitality and vigor.

- <u>Implications for Lifespan and Health Span</u>

They are the pioneers of growth in working out as to how long-lived man may be while mimicking caloric restriction and relevant effects cannot be limited only towards lifespan extension peeking through health span and vigor proliferation. As mediators of fundamental metabolic pathways that implicate cellular processes that underlie senescence; caloric restriction mimetics stand out as prologues to age-resistant resilience paving means of cancelling physiological features driving aging whereby the boundaries will be shifted in medical science.

At the heart of these potential for transformation lies their ability to conduct physiological adaptations that lifted themselves and slid beyond the boundaries of biological age. These interventions impart the inflammatory spark by which protection from aging pathologies are initiated, igniting an inferno of mitochondrial biogenesis that feeds the fires of cellular energy utilization that power organisms. Through enhancement of mitochondrial functioning and resilience, caloric restriction mimetics provide cells with adequate metabolic energy to work it through as long possible in a fight against the devastating effects caused by aging.

In addition, caloric restriction mimetics have a great impact on the complex choreography of glucose metabolism, coordinating fundamental positions between insulin sensitivity polarity glycolytic flux cells energetic state. Fusing the terms control, interventions and metabolism as opposed to 'enable by interventions', One needs to capitalize on modulation of key metabolic regulators such as AMP- activated protein kinase (AMPK) and sirtuin. This way provides individuals with an equipment known as a gift of resilience that allows them an opportunity to enjoy flexibility in met

Additionally, the anti-inflammatory mechanisms of calorie restriction mimetics are a torch's end in an era plagued with chronic disease as it puts out the fire surrounding systemic inflammation that lays like a burning match igniting age-related pathology. Through dampening the madness of pro-inflammatory cytokines and oxidative stressors, these interventions build a fortress of resilience that ensures bunches of cells embrace years within their savable premises.

In essence, the benefits that come beyond the sphere of molecular biology are bound to appear in real-life practice. The effects of caloric restriction mimetics are demonstrated on the paths of cognition, as well in bypasses leading to cardiovascular health improvement – not limited to scattering across a multitude of lab assays and clinical trials. People taking caloric restriction mimetics may discover themselves furnished with wholly unique freshness as the mist of exhaustion is lifted and warm fire in the intens2heart burns back on its energizing.

Furthermore, the anticipated synergism between CRM and congruent measures, including work-out regimes and dietary changes introduces a fundamental transmutation in quest for healthiness and longevity. In this context, it is within the bounds that individuals may weave together different strands of lifestyle interventions in a tapestry of well-being that goes beyond the norms of common sense; because by using all aspects such as dietary approach, physical fitness and pharmacology they are able develop a unified course to healthy life.

Amid the crucible of scientific scrutiny, the vision of caloric restriction mimetics holds sparkling promise among researchers trying to unlock ageless vitality and vivacity. With this unification of molecular biology, pharmacology and translational medicine once more profit from dreaming to work toward that elusive horizon where we understand humans have a new and fresh definition of health through longevity which is life with sparkle, charm and excitement.

To conclude, mimicking caloric restriction embraces a paradigm shift in study as it is the prevalent possibility based on scientific data of longer life and better health. By the unveiling and describing pharmacological factors that mimic metabolic physiology responses of caloric restriction, researchers bring previously untapped opportunities to mitigate age-related decline by supporting an optimal condition throughout aging.

As our understanding of the underlying mechanisms continues to evolve, the development of novel caloric restriction mimetics holds tremendous potential to revolutionize preventive and therapeutic strategies for age-related diseases, paving the way for a future where individuals can not only live longer but also enjoy healthier and more fulfilling lives.

4.4. Practical Applications and Potential Side Effects of Rapamycin Therapy

In the world of longevity science and efforts to improve the healthspan of mankind, Rapamycin has become a viable medicinal substance. Rapamycin was originally designed as an immunosuppressant, but it works in a unique way which makes this antifungal medication popular for the usage in developing interventions aimed at impeding aging and preventing such conditions as cancer, cardiovascular diseases which are regarded signs of aging. In this section, the pragmatic concerns of Rapamycin therapy are analyzed together with its contraindications.

- ## Anti-Aging and Healthspan Extension:

Sweeping away from the idea of aging and its many ailments, scientists have turned their attention towards Rapamycin therapy. This pharmacologically active compound has been reported as one of the potential interventions for promoting longer healthspan and delaying the senescence-related disorders. Its mode of action is centered on the modulation of the mechanistic target of rapamycin (mTOR) pathway, a key regulator of metabolic processes known to be relevant in aging and lifespan.

The basis of Rapamycin's anti-aging properties can be traced down to preclinical studies carried out on various model organisms, from yeast to mammals. All these investigations have shown that Rapamycin treatment can lead to deep effects produced by biological aging. The underlying mechanism of this drug consists in its ability to block the mTOR pathway, the core signaling pathway that coordinates information about nutrient and energy status with cellular growth, metabolism, and aging processes.

One of the basic similarities observed between Rapamycin treatment and other longevity-promoting interventions such as caloric restriction is their capability to actively reduce the effect of mTOR pathway. Although it is well established that caloric restriction reduces mTOR activity, this biological event contributes at least in part to the multiple beneficial effects of this dietary regimen which includes longevity enhancement and improved healthspan across many species. Likewise, Rapamycin has its anti-aging prospects by mimicking the metabolism and cellular events emulated by caloric restriction, but through drug action.

The experiments show the practical side of Rapamycin therapy, which clearly goes beyond theoretical reasoning. Research has revealed numerous benefits of Rapamycin administration that were observed in different animal models, including healthy aging. These include improved metabolic homeostasis, better immunological function, decreased risk for age-related pathologies in cancer and neurodegenerative diseases, even preserved cognitive function into advanced age.

The idea of Rapamycin as a means for promoting healthy aging among people seems to be attracting, especially because of its long history for safe use in Transplant medicine and cancer therapy. On the one side, humanizing Rapamycin's anti-aging potential from animal models to human populations is a work in progress but initial clinical trials and observational studies provide optimistic clues of its effectiveness and safety.

Notably, a pioneering program that has been conducted is the TAME (Targeting Aging with Metformin) trial which was a landmark research project that sought to determine how metformin—a commonly prescribed antidiabetic agent known for potential anti-aging properties—could postpone the onset of age-related diseases. Though Rapamycin is not a main focus area of the TAME trial, its incorporation into future trials that will evaluate multi-modal interventions in healthy aging research carries tremendous potential.

Research of Rapamycin-based interventions for the healthy aging is not without difficulties to consider. But this is just the tip of the iceberg; a primary problem that needs to be addressed concerns the issues raised by balancing potential benefits from improving healthspan against risk for adverse effects and unintended consequences following long-term treatment with Rapamycin. Although one can say that the safety of Rapamycin is relatively well-established in short term therapy, we still need research to answer some questions such as optimum dosing regimen and duration of treatment as well as potential side effects like immunosuppression and metabolic derangement.

The ramification of ageing as a multi-factorial process requires molecular explanations related to the pathways and biological processes influencing decline due to aging. While mTOR pathway can be considered as one possible target of therapeutic intervention, it is merely the part of a system consisting of various interrelated pathways implicated in aging and longevity. Further research in this field may allow us to understand the complex interplay between these pathways that would reveal targeted and viable options for healthy aging.

Rapamycin therapy stands at the forefront of efforts to extend healthspan and mitigate the effects of aging on human health. By targeting the mTOR pathway, Rapamycin mimics the effects of caloric restriction and triggers cellular processes associated with increased lifespan and improved health.

While challenges and uncertainties remain, the growing body of evidence supporting Rapamycin's anti-aging potential underscores its promise as a transformative intervention in the pursuit of healthy aging for all.

- ## **Immunosuppression in Organ Transplantation:**

Organ transplantation constitutes one of the milestones in the history of modern medicine as it provides patients with organic pathology with a chance at better life and prolonged living. Nevertheless, despite the numerous possibilities for transplantation, the body's immune system is only too often capable of obstructing this success by treating the grafted cells as invaders and provoking a vehement rejection response. The basis of transplant medicine is the use of immunosuppressive therapy which works by modulating the immune system and stopping the graft rejection. In addition to the plethora of immunosuppressive agents, Rapamycin stands out from the rest owing to its remarkable potency as a suppressor and unusual anti-immune mechanisms.

Subsequently, after initially being identified as an antifungal agent, rapamycin quickly demonstrated its effectiveness as an immunosuppressant working especially through the process of transplant organization. In contrast to direct T-cell activation, Rapamycin acts indirectly downstream specifically inhibiting growth cytokine regulation and cellular proliferation. Its mechanism of action involves the mTOR signaling pathway inhibition, which is a vital element that shuts significant metabolic processes necessary for immune activation and proliferation.

The blanket of immunosuppression, which is produced by Rapamycin goes far beyond just the role in T-cell inhibition. It also has anti-angiogenic effects that may prevent the necessary blood supply for tumor expansion thus decreasing risk for malignancies after transplantation. Besides, Rapamycin favors the growth of regulatory T cells (Tregs) and enhances dendritic cell functions ensuring immune tolerance maintaining the graft viability over time.

The Combination therapy approach involving Rapamycin has shown a lot of synergy between the drugs used in practice. Combination of Rapamycin with CNIs or other immunosuppressants enables lower individual potencies of the drugs; this helps avoid overdosing and toxicity, yet efficacy of the combination stay high. These mixtures have led a reformation in transplant medicine, leading to improved results and the elimination of rejection incidence.

Though effective the use of Rapamycin is also difficult. To manage care of patients about to undergo these drugs, one needs to consider that its action occurs at a very late stage besides having the potential for adverse side effects such as hyperlipidemia and impaired wound healing. In addition, current research aims at interpreting the mysteries behind immune regulation as well as personalized immunosuppression taking an individual patient's profile into consideration.

Rapamycin with its immunosuppressive action has changed the prospects of organ transplantation, allowing multidimensional modification of immune activity and graft survival. Of significance, its special process of action alongside immunological tolerance has converted transplantation from a dangerous task to some kind of regular and life-saving practice.

With the progress of research and the improvement of our immunosuppression knowledge, it can be concluded that Rapamycin will play more important role in transplantation process and influence patients' future. In the unstoppable race for better transplantation results, people are keeping Rapamycin as a signal of hope referring to the future where organ transplantation becomes not just an alternative but a remedy.

- **Cancer Therapy:**

There are no grounds for slowdown in their efforts to search unceasingly for new approaches emerging in the field of cancer therapy,directed at definite molecular mechanisms. Within these potential alternatives, the group of rapamycin and its analogs combined as rapalogs has emerged as an agent that could potentially change life in favor of addressing cancer. These anti-tumor compounds are effective, because of their inhibitory activity towards malfunctioning mTOR signaling pathways as the primary regulators in the development of numerous cancer types.

However, clinical trials of rapamycin and rapalogs as a cancer therapeutic strategy have received support in managing cancers such as renal cell carcinoma and mantle cell lymphoma through stringent research endeavors, marking the dawn of the modern management era.

Understanding mTOR Signaling:

The development and progression of cancer are based on the disruption of signaling systems necessary for growth, proliferation, and cell survival. A relevant pathway for this example is the mechanistic target of rapamycin (mTOR) signaling, which involves directing cellular responses to various stimuli; these include nutrient availability, growth factors and cellular stress.

The prototypical feature of diverse cancers is dysregulated mTOR signaling activation triggering tumor cell homeostasis, driving uncontrolled growth and survival as well as conferring resistance to classical cytotoxic drugs.

Rapamycin and Rapalogs: Mechanism of Action:

Macrolide antibiotic, rapamycin was initially identified use in Easter Island soil sample for Its anti- tumor activity by virtue of Inhibiting mTORC1. By going into complex with FK506-binding protein 12 (FKBP12), rapamycin inhibits mTORC1 only and that too selectively. In addition to rapamycin, researchers have designed a number of analogs named as rapalogs in order to overcome its some limitations such as shortcomings associated with pharmacokinetics and lesser inhibitory activity on mTOR.

Clinical Efficacy in Renal Cell Carcinoma:

The clinical picture of renal cell carcinoma (RCC) is rather complicated and associated with significant limitations due to the lack of appropriate treatment in the case of advanced-stage disease. Nevertheless, with the advent of the targeted therapies that is rapamycin and rapalogs this has revolutionized the management of RCC. The effects of rapalogs on RCC patients have been extremely promising in clinical trial settings with data showing a significant increase to progression-free survival and overall survival rates. Rapalogs provide a pin spot of hope in that they stunt mTOR-mediated pathways with regard to tumor growth and angiogenesis for RCC patients; they reduce the morbidity associated with tumor burden, resulting in significant benefits both clinically and on quality of life.

Advances in Mantle Cell Lymphoma Treatment:

The most serious therapeutic challenges have been associated with mantle cell lymphoma (MCL), a type of non-Hodgkin lymphoma that overexpresses cyclin D1 and whose hallmark is the disease's invasive nature and recurrences. This is also true for rapamycin and rapalogs which are exciting new therapeutic agents. Preclinical studies revealed the potential efficacy of rapamycin in inducing cell cycle arrest and apoptosis on MCL cells. In addition, clinical trials involving combinations of rapalogs with standard chemotherapy or new agents have yielded promising results that emphasize the therapeutic potential of rapamycin-based treatments in improving patient outcomes from MCL.

Challenges and Future Directions:

Notwithstanding the impressive strides that have been recorded in tapping into rapamycin and rapalogs with anticancer properties, there are several challenges as discussed below. Several formidable challenges arise in their clinical implementation that include resistance mechanisms, off-target effects and dose-limiting toxicities. In addition, the best arrangement and integration algorithms with current treatments need also to be investigated in future so as to achieve optimum efficacy and minimal side effects. Further innovative research opportunities should strive to discover the intricate interdependence between mTOR signaling and other oncogenic pathways that could spark more precision-targeted therapies adapted to tumor specificity.

- **Neuroprotection and Neurological Disorders:**

Alzheimer's disease, Parkinson's disease and Traumatic brain injury are descriptions of their respective pathologies which cause neuronal dysfunction causing cognitive and motor impairment. Although this particular compound is primarily famous for its immunosuppressive properties and relationship in transplant medicine it has prompted a lot of curiosity due to potential results on different neurological diseases.

Understanding Neuroprotection and Neurological Disorders

Neuroprotection refers to methods conducted to maintain the neuronal structure and function, which help in preventing neurodegeneration and brain disorders. Alzheimer's disease is a gradually degrading mental illness that leads to loss of neurons and affects millions of victims globally. Thus, Parkinson's disease featuring dopaminergic degeneration of neurons is characterized by motor incapacities and intellectual deterioration. Traumatic brain injury, an outcome of head trauma results in permanent neurological monadic impairment affecting the cognitive and motor processes.

Rapamycin: Mechanisms of Action and Neuroprotective Effects

The mode of action of Rapamycin is that through modulation of the mechanistic target of rapamycin (mTOR) signal pathway, a vital actor which regulates cellular processes like growth, metabolism and autophagy. Several neurological disorders have been associated with the inhibition of the mTOR signaling pathway. Several mechanisms serve to achieve the neuroprotection by Rapamycin upon its inhibition of mTOR.

Firstly, neuroinflammation is the major contributor to pathogenesis of neurological disorders. The neuroinflammatory mediators are significantly regressed by the application of rapamycin, as depiction shows an attenuation in microglia and astrocyte activation. This ant-inflammatory action inhibits neuronal damage and maintains intellectual activity. Another thing is that Rapamycin helps the neuron survive by inhibiting apoptotic pathways and increasing cellular tolerance to stressors. It regulates the ratio of cell death and life and so, maintains neuronal integrity despite pathological challenges.

The third aspect that is enhanced by Rapamycin is synaptic plasticity which has a role as it is important for the learning and memory process. It promotes the establishment of new synapses and increases the strength of existing ones, neutralizing the effect of decreased synaptic plasticity characteristic for some neurodegenerative disorders.

Clinical Implications and Therapeutic Potential

Rapamycin promises neuroprotection and this makes it a potent candidate for the treatment of various neurological disorders. In preclinical trials, Rapamycin has shown effectiveness in animal models of Alzheimer's disease, Parkinson's disease and traumatic brain injury. These results support it as a versatile therapeutic agent showing the ability to combat numerous molecular processes of pathological nature that are conducive toward neurological impairment.

In addition, Rapamycin's safety and its well-defined pharmacokinetics as demonstrated by large scale use in transplant medicine assures a good starting point for translation. To date, trials of Rapamycin as potentially efficacious in Alzheimer's disease and traumatic brain injury are ongoing, giving hope for further treatment strategies in these complex conditions.

Challenges and Future Directions

Although rapamycin clearly possesses large potential as a neuroprotective therapy, there are also some challenges in harnessing this approach. There is however need to conduct further studies on the best dosing regimens, adverse and potential side effects and long-term safety considerations. Furthermore, these will elucidate the specific mechanisms behind Rapamycin's neuroprotective effects which will increase our understanding of its therapeutic value but also help develop targeted interventions guided by such actions.

-   **<u>Metabolic Disorders and Obesity:</u>**

Recently, some candidates have been arisen including Rapamycin – an established strong immunosuppressant & mTOR inhibitor that to modulates glucose metabolism and insulin sensitivity. Through exploring its mechanisms and consequences, a gradual narrative is painted that illustrates both the potential benefits and confounding challenges associated with its use.

Underlying Rapamycin's intrigue in the overall shape of things to come is its capacity to reverse the actual disorder between metabolic way that indicate states, for example, diabetes and plumpness. These disorders are significantly linked to the mTOR pathway, which represents a central regulator of cell proliferation and metabolism. Using Scopus, the article indicates that Rapamycin inhibits mTOR producing cellular processes related to glucose uptake, insulin signaling and lipid metabolism as a multidimensional approach towards metabolic dysfunction.

But it is not that simple, as the connection between Rapamycin and metabolic health goes beyond just a correlation. On the contrary, long-term Rapamycin medication may increase metabolic suffering in some patients, reaffirming its dosage and duration as essentials when administered. Despite this, evidence is now emerging that intermittent or short-term utilization of Rapamycin may have the potential to exploit their beneficial effects while averting harmful ones.

Research regarding Rapamycin s effects on glucose metabolism highlight the therapeutic utility of this drug in treating diabetes. The ability of Rapamycin to modulate insulin signaling via targeting GSK3 and Akt, enhances glucose uptake through mTOR complex two thereby improving glycemic control with increased insulin sensitivity. Additionally, its targeted approach towards correcting abnormal lipid metabolism proves valuable in addressing the complex reality of metabolic conditions.

In obesity circles, Rapamycin is moving to the center stage as a metabolic blower. Rapamycin mediates lipid oxidation and an ensuing blockade of adipocyte differentiation that may work as a therapeutic strategy to oppose obesity metabolic disorders. Additionally, its mediating roles on appetite control and calorie burning as well provide pathways for unearthing the novel anti-obesity approaches.

However, translating the efficacy of Rapamycin into clinical practice cannot occur without an appreciation of its dosing schedules and therapeutic approaches. The best dosing regimens should aim to achieve favorable outcomes while at the same time account for minimizing side effects, hence strike a delicate balance between immediate benefits and long-term liabilities. More importantly, factors such as the patient condition and underlying metabolic phenotypes further emphasize the importance of person-specific approaches to treatment.

Apart from the direct impact on metabolic routes, Rapamycin gives larger implications concerning aging and longevity studies. Given its involvement in cellular senescence and longevity pathways, Rapamycin is a prospective anti-aging intervention having bearing on age-related metabolic deterioration. On the other hand, therapies aimed at increasing longevity should be approached with caution as they try to evade the metabolic risks and poor quality of life that comes with increased lifespan.

Understanding in depth the potential of Rapamycin as a therapeutic agent, interdisciplinary collaboration and research innovation become crucial in the process. Using insights from three fields, namely molecular biology, clinical medicine, and systems biology will shed light on the complex relationship between Rapamycin and metabolic homeostasis allowing for personalized treatment approaches based on patient needs.

The capability of rapamycin to regulate glucose metabolism and insulin sensitivity serves as a dynamic approach in treating hectic conditions such as diabetes and obesity. Although obstacles persist in maximizing its therapeutic efficacy and mitigating potential side effects, the nascent field of Rapamycin research presents an opportunity to develop new strategies for addressing the increasing impacts of metabolic disease and requires additional development. As further explorations and partnership continue, Rapamycin may serve as a linchpin in the armory against metabolic diseases promising better treatment outcomes and well-being among millions worldwide.

These practical applications highlight the diverse therapeutic potential of Rapamycin across various medical domains, from anti-aging interventions to cancer therapy and beyond. As research continues to uncover the intricate mechanisms underlying Rapamycin's effects, the development of targeted therapies and personalized treatment approaches holds promise for improving patient outcomes and advancing the field of medicine.

CHAPTER 5
INVESTIGATING METFORMIN

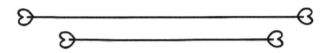

5.1. The Role of Metformin in Managing Type 2 Diabetes

T2DM has been identified as chronic metabolic disorder, since it is characterized by insulin resistance and reduced secretion of insulin with hyperglycemia. As the disorder becomes more and more common worldwide, proper management strategies are essential to control the progression of complications and ensure patients' quality of life. In the range of numerous pharmacological agents that are applied in T2DM treatment therapy, Metformin is recognized as a key drug due to its efficacy and activity profile with multiple mechanisms of actions.

- **<u>Understanding Type 2 Diabetes Mellitus:</u>**

T2DM understanding comprises basic knowledge in comprehending its complicated pathophysiology. Firstly, insulin as a pancreatic hormone plays the central role in this metabolic phenomenon with vital actions concerning glucose homeostasis and energy metabolism. Metabolic alterations and systemic complications will thus ensue following the disrupted intricate balance between insulin production, secretion, and sensitivity typically observed in T2DM individuals.

Firstly, insulin plays the role of facilitating glucose movement from blood into different tissues and cells all over the body. Insulin serves as a crucial facilitator of the binding reaction to cellular receptors, granting glucose access to the cytoplasm where this molecule is either utilized for immediate metabolism or stored atop glycogen reserves. Despite this fact, with regard to T2DM cells become resistant to insulin gradually and therefore this phenomenon termed as insulin resistance.

Insulin resistance, therefore, ultimately changes the nature of responses to glucose metabolism thus leading to poor uptake by cells. As a result, despite sufficient amount of insulin in the blood, the cells cannot react correctly to it-signaling and the blood glucose levels do not normalize; rather higher than acceptable remains an inherent property of T2DM. This process creates the situation in a spiral whereby pancreas is forced to respond by increasing the production of insulin for it to be able to overcome resistance with resultant beta cell exhaustion and impaired secretion.

Additionally, the worsening loss of pancreatic beta-cell function increases the hyperglycemic pathway since inadequate release of insulin adds to tissue utilization disturbance. This dual deficit—resistance to insulin as well as impaired release of insulin—can be regarded a basis for development of T2DM, causing an unstoppable progression towards the disease and its complications.

The impacts of unregulated hyperglycemia are vastly more than raised blood sugar levels. Persistently high glucose levels carry out systemic insults to blood vessels and several organs, causing a range of devastating complications. The major complication in terms of mortality and morbidity in T2DM is cardiovascular complications such as coronary artery, stroke, and peripheral vascular disease.

The negative impacts of hyperglycemia far reaches to the peripheral nervous system leading to diabetic neuropathy that leads to sensory losses, painful sensation and eventually irreversible motor function loss. In the same way, diabetic nephropathy is a common T2DM complication leading to progressive kidney damage that facultatively ends at end stage renal disease requiring dialysis or transplant.

The complex interaction between impaired insulin resistance, insulin secretion dysfunction, and systemic complications demonstrates integrative nature of T2DM making it evident in the necessity to develop comprehensive therapeutic approaches that address both hyperglycemia and its comorbidities. In this regard, pharmacological interventions are of critical importance and help in attaining glycemic control that also reduces the risk of complications.

Metformin, an important player in T2DM management, exploits its beneficial effects mostly by targeting insulin resistance and hepatic glucose production. Humans hyperglycemia due to T2DM is relieved through actions of Metformin alleviating the metabolic derangements that characterize this condition by sensitizing peripheral tissues and suppressing hepatic gluconeogenesis hence improving glucose utilization and reduction of fasting blood

Besides, Metformin provides more cardiovascular benefits than glycemic control when we take lipid profile and endothelial function into consideration, thus highlighting the central position of this oral hypoglycemic in the management of T2DM and its co-morbidities.

A nuanced understanding of T2DM pathophysiology is paramount in guiding effective management strategies aimed at mitigating hyperglycemia and preventing the onset of debilitating complications. Through targeted interventions addressing insulin resistance, impaired insulin secretion, and systemic complications, clinicians can optimize outcomes and enhance the quality of life for individuals living with T2DM.

- **Mechanism of Action of Metformin:**

The metformin, which is entitled the cornerstone of T2DM management due the peculiar mechanism of action that distinct it from conventional antidiabetic drugs. In contrast to beta cell-mediated action of the drugs that increase insulin secretion from the pancreatic cells, Metformin, chemically named as dimethyl-biguanide acts on fundamental mechanisms and pathways involving glucose metabolism and cellular energy regulation.

Among all drug classes for antihyperglycemic agents, one can find a representative of the biguanide class named as Metformin. Its pharmacological implications focus on promoting insulin sensitivity to regulate the hepatic gluconeogenesis that are central issues in T2DM pathology. Interestingly, Metformin's efficacy goes beyond simple glucose-lowering as it triggers a concerted chain of events within the cellular environment that is mediated mainly through the activation of adenosine monophosphate-activated protein kinase (AMPK), an important energy sensor and regulator within a cell.

The essence of Metformin lies in its incredible tendency to create energy through AMPK, the central master metabolic switch that controls many cellular operations. This has the downstream effect of activating AMPK, which in turn sets off a series of reactions that focus on regulating glucose homeostasis. Among its cardinal functions, it aims in increasing the glucose uptake by peripheral tissues mainly skeletal muscles thus enhancing insulin sensitivity. Metformin accelerates the transport of glucose into cells that help in using it efficiently as an energy source, and this contributes to lowering down hyperglycemia thus decreasing insulin resistance.

In addition, metformin has a very powerful inhibitory action on hepatic gluconeogenesis, the complex reaction of liver turning lactate; glycerol and amino acids into glucose. Metformin sets out to address the fundamental cause of fasting blood glucose elevation due to T2DM, by curbing the excessive production of glucose that takes place in the liver. This double approach of increased peripheral glucose consumption and decreased hepatic glucose production also highlights the powerful therapeutic effects of Metformin with its ability to restore euglycemia.

The complexity of Metformin's mechanism is also far from the direct implications of glucose metabolism. AMPK activation, by Metformin, is working a song that has an echo around cellular realms. Specifically, the activity of AMPK leading to mTORC1 suppression points towards Metformin being a potential compound able to regulate cell growth and metabolism. Further, AMPK activation results in alterations in lipid metabolism favoring FFAO and limiting LD synthesis thereby minimizing the dyslipidemia that is common with T2DM.

The therapeutic scope of Metformin goes beyond control of glucose, comprising other metabolic malfunction related to T2DM. Discussed above is the positive effect on body weight primarily because of reduced appetite and mild loss of adiposity, which highlights its potential use as a complementary approach in patients with obesity-induced insulin resistance management. In addition, newer evidence implies the therapeutic effects of Metformin in reducing cardiovascular risk secondary to its reparative processes on endothelial function, inflammation and oxidative stress.

While Metformin shows a deep impact on the course of treatment, it does have its limitations and unwanted outcomes. As for disadvantages, gastrointestinal intolerance associated with nausea, diarrhea and abdominal discomfort is one of the most common side effects that may require dose tittering or adjunctive therapy. Although these complications are rare but severe, this highlights the necessity of extremely careful prescribing practices and most in people with compromise renal function or predisposing factors.

The rise of metformin as first line treatment in T2DM is owed to its base mechanism of action, AMPK activation and modifying important metabolic pathways. Metformin, however, exemplifies a change of paradigm in the management of T2DM by its improvement in insulin sensitivity, inhibition of hepatic glucose production and broad effects on cellular metabolism providing not only glycemic control but also beneficial actions across metabolic and cardiovascular domains. However, judicious monitoring and individualized therapy remain imperative to optimize efficacy and mitigate adverse effects, ensuring that Metformin continues to uphold its stature as a cornerstone in diabetes management.

- **<u>Effects on Lipid Metabolism and Weight:</u>**

As a main stone of T2DM treatment, metformin has distinct effects that are not restricted to glycemic control but encompass lipid regulation and weight management. This understanding is therefore very critical in ensuring that there are informed therapeutic solutions and it is needful to mitigate the cardiovascular risks associated with T2DM.

Lipid metabolism modifying is an essential aspect of Metformin multi-targeting mechanisms. Studies highlight its ability to improve lipid profile, as demonstrated by the decrease both in LDL-C and triglyceride levels. LDL-C and triglycerides respectively high concentrations also represent major risk factors for atherosclerosis and CVD the well-known complications of T2DM. Metformin helps to ameliorate these lipids and they contribute, to a certain degree, towards the decrease of CVD risk burden in influenced people.

Simultaneously, Therapeutic use of Metformin observes slight increases in high density lipoprotein cholesterol (HDL-C), otherwise known as the 'good' cholesterol with anti-atherosclerotic qualities. This staged betterment of lipids parameters through lower LDL-C and triglycerides compared against increased HDL-C may be responsible for the reported improvements in lipid profile during treatment with Metformin.

In addition, weight management affects long-term clinical outcomes and overall health as a result of the influence Metformin exerts on it. While well-known for its glucose lowering efficacy, metformin is considered to aid modest weight reduction or stabilization in individuals affected by T2DM. The exact mechanisms providing these weight-modulating activities are still elusive, however a number of potential factors have received attention.

A hypothetical mechanism involves Metformin-induced reduced appetite, leading to the reduction of caloric consumption and weight-loss as a result. It is important to mention that empirical studies imply that metformin can attenuate appetite hence reducing the food intake leading to weight loss in a susceptible population.

Additionally, the mechanisms through which Metformin regulates weight mainly rely on its insulin-sensitizing effects. It is important in augmenting insulin sensitivity that leads to glucose uptake and utilization by peripheral tissues, hence preventing excess storage of glucose in the body leading to adiposity. As a result, the ancillary benefits of weight management restored through insulin sensitivity in T2DM that Metformin confers further support its role as a key therapy in treatment.

The next emerging evidence demonstrates the crucial role of gut microbiota modulation as a mechanism by which metabolic effects, including weight regulation are mediated by interventions with Metformin. Changes in composition of gut microbiota by metformin can have further functional consequences, affecting absorption of nutrients, calorigenic responses and host physiology.

Changes in the composition of GI microbiota caused by Metformin therapy may increase metabolically advantages that make weight loss or stabilization possible for susceptible persons.

In addition, the relationship between Metformin and gut microbiota reflects the delicate balance between host physiology and microbial ecology, unlocking new horizons for treatment of metabolic comorbidity via synergistic partner therapy.

Taken together, the favorable impact of metformin on lipid metabolism and weight loss is key to its central role in comprehensive management or control of T2DM. Metformin represents a pinnacle of the integrative pharmacotherapy ideal by targeting several different components of metabolic deregulation in T2DM pathophysiology.

Nevertheless, the complex interdependency between Metformin, lipid metabolism and weight control require continued efforts in research on its underlying mechanisms. Understanding the precise molecular mechanisms controlling Metformin's metabolic impact will importantly inform the future refinement of therapeutic strategies and realization of patient optimization outcomes in the management of T2DM.

Metformin's profound impact on lipid metabolism and weight regulation transcends its conventional role as a glucose-lowering agent, emblematic of its status as a cornerstone therapy in T2DM management. By modulating lipid profiles, promoting weight loss or stabilization, and mitigating cardiovascular risk burden, Metformin embodies a quintessential therapeutic arsenal in the armamentarium against T2DM and its associated complications.

- **Clinical Efficacy and Safety Profile:**

Metformin is a powerful type 2 antidiabetic agent and has been found to be very effective on clinical trials as well as real-life studies in the management of type, thus becoming the backbone in the treatment of T2DM. It has been shown to possess high efficacy and safety profile, and this has placed it at a vantage position as an effective first-line therapy whether used alone or in isolation with other hypoglycemic agents. This chapter discusses the clinical effectiveness and safety implications regarding Metformin in the overcome T2DM.

Clinical Efficacy:

The ability of metformin in glycemic control has been proven by several clinical trials and observational observation. As a biguanide, Metformin mostly functions through the reduction of hepatic glucose production, enhanced peripheral glucose uptake as well as improved insulin sensitivity. These functions help it to be effective in reducing blood glucose.

In the clinical settings, Metformin has shown remarkable results toward elimination of hemoglobin A1c (HbA1c), fasting plasma glucose (FPG) and postprandial glucose levels. In addition, it continued to be effective for a long duration of time which made it an irreplaceable quality in the management of T2DM.

The farthest limits of metformin's versatility demonstrate the fact that it should not be a monotherapy. It works effectively with a range of other anti-diabetic drugs like sulfonylureas, DPP-4 inhibitors and SGLT2 that are chosen depending on distinct patient needs seeking glycemic goals. The flexibility of this technique points to the role it plays in an integrated approach to T2DM management.

Safety Profile:

Metformin's safety profile is quite favorable overall, its adverse effects rarely occur. The most common side effects of treatment include such gastrointestinal symptoms as nausea, diarrhea or abdominal discomfort. Nevertheless, these issues tend to decrease as the treatment goes on or if dosage could be altered, and so with that alone they do little or nothing to affect patient compliance or quality of life.

Although the use of Metformin is considered to be well-tolerated by most patients, there are some extremely rare but serious complications that should not be neglected. Regardless of infrequence, lactic acidosis is considered a severe adverse effect resulted from Metformin intake. This complication is potentiated in patients with renal impairment or underlying predispositions and thus must be meticulously prescribed and, importantly, tracked for renal function routinely.

Metformin plays a key clinical role in the management of T2DM, given its activity and high levels of safety. It provides significant advantages as a therapy used initially in glycemic control and cardiovascular risk reduction. Complementary efficacy with other antidiabetic agents highlights its multidimensional nature and importance of its use in personalized regimes.

But rules concerning the rare but severe side effects of Metformin are mandated for clinicians, particularly on lactic acidosis in patients with renal deficiency. As healthcare providers can enhance patient outcomes by balancing therapy benefits with associated harms, they should ensure responsive utilization of Metformin in T2DM treatment.

Overall, a conceptual understanding of the clinical effectiveness and safety aspects underpinning Metformin enables clinicians to make informed decisions when managing T2DM so as improve patient care and ensure long-term results.

5.2.   Activation of AMPK: Metabolic Effects and Implications for Aging

Within the context of aging, one vital mechanism critically affecting metabolism is the activation of adenosine monophosphate-activated protein kinase (AMPK), which plays an essential role. The main role of AMPK is to control cellular energy balance and it acts as the key regulator in many metabolic pathways. This paper discusses the complex mechanisms by which AMPK activation takes place, its metabolic implications and its importance in aging process.

AMP-activated protein kinase (AMPK) serves as a pivotal regulator of cellular energy homeostasis, orchestrating adaptive responses to fluctuations in energy availability and demand. Its activation represents a sophisticated mechanism by which cells sense and respond to alterations in the intracellular energy state.

This discussion elucidates the fundamental principles underlying AMPK activation, encompassing its triggers, signaling pathways, and physiological implications.

- ## **Metabolic Effects of AMPK Activation**

Metabolic homeostasis is considered one of the basic functional characteristics of a cell, because life is only possible with constant metabolism and in response to changing environmental signals. Adenosine monophosphate-activated protein kinase (AMPK), a master regulator which senses and coordinates cellular energy status plays at the core of this delicate regulatory network. Upon initiation, AMPK conducts a series of metabolic responses tailored towards restoring the energy equilibrium while promoting cell resistance and hence cell survival and functions.

Another major function of AMPK enation is to adjust cellular metabolism to cope with changing need levels for energy. AMPK is activated by phosphorylation and the allosteric regulation that takes place when cellular energy levels are low, such as during increased energy utilization or deficiency of nutrients. When it is activated, AMPK induces a chain of adaptive reactions that are aimed to maintain energy homeostasis and cell survival.

A central pathway which AMPK mediates in energy homeostasis is the induction of catabolic routes that produce adenosine triphosphate (ATP), the main currency of cellular energy. Activation of AMPK in skeletal muscle promotes glucose uptake and glycolysis to allow the generation of ATP from glucose through phosphorylation, responding to the increasing demand for energy due to enhanced metabolic activity. AMPK increases glucose consumption to promote adequate cellular ATP, which provides for essential cellular processes and maintains functional cell structure.

In addition to accelerating glucose metabolism, activation of AMPK enhances fatty acid oxidation and mitochondrial biogenesis that increases the ability of cells to burn the second energy source. AMPK stimulates mitochondrial function and oxidative metabolism, enabling cells to efficiently oxidize fatty acids for the synthesis of ATP in a further boosting cellular energy production. This metabolic flexibility enables cells to respond to the external adjustments in nutrient supply and masked conditions of metabolism, thereby ensuring energy homeostasis and cellular survival.

In addition to this, the activation of AMPK is a key mechanism in preventing metabolic stress and oxidative damage. In times of metabolic imbalance i.e nutrient excess and alleviating cellular stress when there is oxidative stress, activation of AMPK would help to modulate various metabolic pathways. For instance, AMPK inhibits processes that are energy costly by their anabolic nature including protein and lipid synthesis; thus conserving energy resources directing metabolism towards ATP producing pathways.

Additionally, AMPK-activation increases intracellular antioxidant defenses and facilitates compensatory removal of defective organelles via autophagy, leading to a reduction in oxidative damage and preservation of cellular functionality. Through the coordination of the adaptive responses, AMPK participates in maintaining cellular homeostasis and preventing metabolic disorder as well as disease.

One way or another, the metabolic effects of AMPK activation goes beyond single cell to impact the whole-body metabolism and energy balance. Other than controlling metabolism in the cell, AMPK therefore serves central organizer of signals from different tissues and organs such as liver, adipose tissue, and brain. By responding to systemic status, AMPK co-ordinates metabolic responses between tissues ensuring that supply of energy matches demand.

In addition, AMPK signaling dysfunction is associated with metabolic disorders like obesity, type 2 diabetes as well as cardiovascular disease. AMPK activating pharmacological agents have exhibited tremendous therapeutic effectiveness for these conditions, suggesting the need to better understand all manner of control functions that governs AMPK expression.

AMPK activation performs multiple functions on cell metabolism and represents the adaptive mechanisms that act to re-establish balance of energy and improve resistance. AMPK also manages glucose and fatty acid metabolism, improves mitochondrial function, and inhibits oxidative stress to maintain cellular homeostasis that prevents the onset of metabolic dysfunction. The knowledge about the metabolic processes that are modified upon AMPK activation is crucial for understanding pathogenesis as well as for proposing possible therapeutic modalities.

- **Implications for Aging**

The aging process is also associated with the reduced functional capacity of the cells and loss of integrity tissue, as well as high predisposition for a range of age-related diseases. The entire process of ageing involves changes to the cellular energy metabolism, which is a significant factor in determining the resistance capacity and overall organismal health by focusing on key body systems. The stimulation of AMPK, a major transcriptional control point for cellular energy levels that is thought to become dysregulated during aging, also impacts age-related metabolism by altering fundamental metabolic pathways and combatting age-associated abnormalities.

This is because, with age, the capacity of energy production by cells deteriorates and thus designated to negative metabolism leftovers. This metabolic inefficiency is a key factor of the development and aggravation of age-related pathologies, such as cardiovascular disease, neurodegenerative disorders or metabolic syndrome. Activating AMPK is undoubtedly a progressive therapeutic approach that may help to combat age-related metabolic decline and promote healthy aging by increasing mitochondrial function and oxidative metabolism.

The Mitochondria, the cells energy source, takes part in much of cellular ATP production and homeostasis. As a person ages, mitochondria functions start deteriorating and this leads to enhanced oxidative stress and impaired mitochondrial function. Studies have demonstrated that AMPK activation strengthens mitochondrial biogenesis and augments mitochondrial function by improving their oxidative capacity and their impairment with oxidants. The activation of AMPK prevents damage to mitochondrial integrity thus ensuring the maintenance of energy balance and prevention of the deleterious effects caused by metabolic decline associated with aging.

Additionally, AMPK activation leads to anti-inflammatory effects due to the fact that it inhibits pro-inflammatory pathways hence suppressing the production of inflammatory mediators seen in chronic diseases associated with aging. Chronic inflammation is considered one of the most typical manifestations of aging, and it associates with various conditions associated with agedness such as cardiovascular disease, diabetes, and neurodegenerative disorders. Through its capacity to reduce the inflammation chronic AMPK activation may play a role in features that impede the age-related pathologies and also influences healthy living long.

In addition, AMPK activation can also improve cellular mechanisms of resistance to stress such as autophagy and proteostasis that help to maintain intracellular homeostasis through clearance of damaged proteins and organelles. One of the cellular processes responsible for autophagy, degradation and recycling of cellular components decreases with age which leads to accumulation of the dysfunctional organelles as well as protein aggregates anywhere in older age people and those who also indulge themselves into diseases that occur during old age. One of the mechanisms that AMPK activation promotes autophagy from is by activating essential regulators of autophagy, helping in improving cell quality control and tissue homeostasis.

Apart from its effect on modulating cellular metabolism and inflammation, the activation of AMPK has also potential benefits in cognitive impairment associated with aging along with neurodegenerative diseases. Emerging data support that AMPK activation may be protective against neuronal damage and cognitive declines as a result of its neurogenesis, synaptic plasticity, and neuronal survivals. Increased brain energy metabolism and decreased oxidative stress mediated by AMPK activation may contribute to the preservation of cognitive integrity during aging, and protect against age-related neurodegeneration as demonstrated with Parkinson's disease, for example.

Furthermore, the metabolic impacts of AMPK activation pose great implications for aging process improvement due to mitochondrial function and inflammation reduction as well as cellular stress resistance mechanisms promotion. The designation of key metabolic signaling pathways as targets for AMPK activation can be considered one of the promising therapeutic approaches to improve healthy aging and prevent age-associated diseases. Additional studies are also needed to understand completely the benefits of AMPK activation can be used effectively for enhancing longevity and retaining healthspan in aged populations.

In brief, the activation of AMPK is a primary mechanism with powerful metabolic connotations and deep implications in aging development. Through s coordination of adaptive reactions to the changes in the cellular energy status AMPK activation represents one of central functions for metabolic homeostasis together with strengthening of cell resistance toward metabolic challenges. Further, AMPK activation shows therapeutic prospects for age-related metabolic disorders and chronic diseases suggesting new intervention approaches that facilitate healthy aging with an extended life span. New discoveries about these mechanisms and how this molecule affects aging processes will no doubt uncover previously unknown ways to improve health and longevity in the future.

5.3. Reducing Inflammation and Oxidative Stress: Mechanisms Underlying Longevity Benefits

Throughout the efforts to lengthen human lifespan and enhance overall health, researchers have placed a growing emphasis on the delicate balance between inflammation, oxidative stress, and longevity. Both inflammations, a biological reaction thought to be associated with damage and oxidative stress involving an imbalance between free radicals and antioxidants, are crucial determinants underlying the aging process and age-related diseases. It is also promising that the mechanisms of how inflammation and oxidative stresses are associated with a lifespan promise more novel therapeutic treatments and lifestyle applications in aging retardation.

- **The Role of Chronic Inflammation in Aging**

The distinguishing condition of persistent inflammation, known as "inflammaging," has taken pride in advancement as a popular phenomenon vital for the internal workings for the delicate age mechanics. It signifies in many cases a landmark feature of age-related diseases and goes from cardiovascular poisonous to neurodegenerative disorder, malignancy. In this chapter, the authors examine a detailed and complex relationship between chronic inflammation and aging, explaining cellular mechanisms, molecular routes, and clinical implications of this sophisticated interaction.

Chronic inflammation consists of an intensive cascade of cellular pathways directed by cytokines, especially interleukin-6 (IL- 6) and tumor nerve factor alpha (TNF-alpha). These cytokines were identified to function as main conductor in inflaming and perpetuating responses in tissues and organs. Inflammation is a vital natural response to invasions that intent to kill pathogens, prevent tissue injury and maintain homeostasis whenever disrupted by the same activities, thus detrimental consequences kick starts with chronic inflammatory activities in aging.

However, chronic inflammation in the environment of a cell exerts more severe effects causing oxidative stress and ultimately leading to nuclear damage by increasing the process rate of apoptosis that is now termed 'cellular senescence' or biological aging. However, under continued bombardment by ROS generated during inflammatory processes the growth integrity is broken down and the mitochondria degenerates to a point where not even the DNA of these cells can escape. As a result, cells experience a slow decline that includes loss capacity and impoverishing regenerative capability – age related characteristics of an aged tissue.

Additionally, chronic inflammation produces a hostile cultivation environment that is suitable for the commencement as well as continuance of age associated disorders. In vascular field, inflammatory cytokines have an effect of endothelial dysfunction that helps atherosclerotic plaque creation and places people who are on the verge of a myocardial infarction or stroke. Likewise, in the brain, neuroinflammation initiates neuronal injury and synapse depletion causing an environment for neurodegenerative disorders such as Alzheimer's and Parkinson's diseases.

In addition, the complex interplay between chronic inflammation and cancer due to the very multi-layered nature of cancer. Tumorigenesis becomes intensified by inflammatory mediators in developing a pro-proliferative state, endorsing angiogenesis and escaping immune surveillance. Additionally, chronic inflammation causes mutations of genes and epigenetic changes, promoting the malignant transformation of cells and ensuring selective information for cancerous clones. Therefore, the integration of chronic inflammation and cancer shows that it stands as the central figure in defining aging and how disease development evolves.

Prolonged inflammation affects clinical outcomes and life span, clinical observations support this intensely. Inflammatory markers, CRP and IL-6 with elevated circulating levels are prognostic indicators of poor myocardial events as well as mortality in a diseased age population. Additionally, therapeutic approaches directed at inflammatory pathways have indicated potential to alleviate age-related morbidities as well as increase healthspan. Inflammatory burden can be reduced and the harmful effects of inflammaging counteract with lifestyle modifications such as physical activity, diets loaded with antioxidants, or even behavioral changes to reduce stress.

With this in mind, chronic inflammation emerges as a main character on the story unraveling aging by influencing cellular senescence, tissue homoeostasis and susceptibility. The complex interplay between telomere, oxidative stress, genomic instability and its role in immune dysregulation highlights the multifaceted nature of this phenomenon that defines aging and age-related disease. Therefore, elucidation of the molecular mechanisms underlying chronic inflammation has a great potential in identifying prospective novel therapeutic approaches and interventional strategies aimed at promoting healthy ageing and increasing healthspan. By adopting an integrative approach that incorporates lifestyle management, pharmacological interventions and precision medicine practices is the sure way of reducing inflammaging pressure and building a healthy aging population.

- **<u>Oxidative Stress: The Double-Edged Sword of Aging</u>**

Oxidative stress becomes a critical factor in aging, characterized by its duality: on one hand, oxidative stress is a profound requirement for cellular function whose purpose is necessary to enable cells' vital activities; on the other hand, it marks the start of cell destruction. This condition evolves from the precarious equilibrium that prevails between ROS and antioxidant defense system of the body. Although ROS play a substantive role in cellular signaling and homeostasis, unrestricted accrual of these presumably leads to the buildup of harmful substances, which contribute largely to aging and create an environment that readily forms age-related diseases. This inquiry elucidates the delicate dynamic between oxidative stress and aging process, revealing its intricacies and meaning.

The Nature of Oxidative Stress: Implicit value of oxidative stress is a result of ROS overcome and body's capability to counter these ROS generation. ROS includes many compounds like superoxide radicals, hydrogen peroxide and hydroxyl free-radicals ROS is the byproduct of cellular metabolism as well as they have girl's crucial roles in signaling pathways. On the other hand, oxidative stress results from greater generation of ROS that is above and beyond what endogenous antioxidant mechanisms can achieve and thus promote an environment icy sustaining cellular damage.

ROS-Mediated Damage and Aging: The deleterious effects of oxidative stress reverberate across various cellular components, culminating in the hallmark features of aging. Proteins, the workhorses of cellular function, fall prey to oxidative modifications, compromising their structural integrity and functional efficacy. Lipids, crucial constituents of cellular membranes, succumb to peroxidation, perturbing membrane fluidity and permeability. DNA, the custodian of genetic information, suffers oxidative lesions, undermining genomic stability and fidelity. Collectively, these assaults contribute to the gradual deterioration of cellular machinery, heralding the onset of aging.

Age-Related Pathologies and Oxidative Stress: The insidious effects of cumulative oxidative stress extend beyond the realm of cellular aging, predisposing individuals to a spectrum of age-related pathologies. Cardiovascular disease, a leading cause of mortality worldwide, manifests in part due to oxidative modification of lipids and proteins within vascular endothelial cells, culminating in endothelial dysfunction and atherosclerosis. Neurodegenerative disorders, typified by Alzheimer's and Parkinson's diseases, showcase a predilection for regions of heightened oxidative stress, exacerbating neuronal damage and cognitive decline. Metabolic disorders, including diabetes mellitus and obesity, bear witness to the dysregulation of cellular redox homeostasis, engendering insulin resistance and aberrant lipid metabolism. Thus, oxidative stress emerges as a common denominator underlying the pathogenesis of diverse age-related ailments.

Counteracting Oxidative Stress: The Role of Antioxidants: In the battle against oxidative stress, antioxidants stand as stalwart defenders, scavenging ROS and restoring redox equilibrium. Endogenous antioxidants, comprising enzymatic systems such as superoxide dismutase, catalase, and glutathione peroxidase, orchestrate a coordinated defense against oxidative insults. Exogenous antioxidants, derived from dietary sources such as vitamins C and E, bolster endogenous defenses, augmenting the cellular armamentarium against oxidative stress. Moreover, lifestyle modifications, including regular physical activity and prudent dietary choices, confer additional resilience against oxidative damage, underscoring the multifaceted nature of antioxidant strategies.

Thus, the physiology of oxidation is seen to be vitally essential as a participant in aging, but when it becomes so excessive and uncontrolled that irreparable damage results – snaps into being and remains one of pathological necessity. Reactive oxygen species play an essential role in signal transduction and cellular functioning, though when left unchecked ROS proliferation leads to a series of pathological outcomes that include 'ageing' and increased likelihood of age-associated disease conditions. By delving into the complex nature of reactive oxidation and its consequences we open a window to interventions and countermeasures, leveraging antioxidant defense mechanisms as well as supportive living practices to reinforce cellular resilience relative to time. Thus, oxidative stress also works as an index of a significant reminder as we age because the cyclical and counteracting nature based on human biology represents such the continuance.

- ## Longevity Benefits of Reducing Inflammation and Oxidative Stress

The encouragement of the inexorable ambition to enlarge human life and improve overall health by plunging into efforts, research has more or less turned its attention towards grips with chronic inflammation and oxidative stress as key variables implicated in aging and disease progression. Chronic inflammatory state and oxidative stress, result of an imbalance between free radicals and antioxidants, establish a relationship to their mutual interdependence, significant contributing factors that influence the aging process.

An enormous variety of approaches to suppress inflammation oxidative stress has been revealed by scientific investigations as prerequisites for the possible benefits in extending longevity and appropriate retention of health span. A renowned strategy includes food diet controls, focusing on the enrichment of anti-inflammatory nutrients that are rich in antioxidants which involves eating fruits vegetables nuts and fatty fish. These dietary factors contribute adequate and necessary nutrients in addition to bioactive compounds so as to quench free radicals, which reduce the inflammation process that may occur within the body.

In addition, studies have shown that regular physical exercise can turn out to be a powerful mediator of inflammation and oxidative stress. In addition to improving cardiovascular fitness and muscle power, exercise also has tremendous anti-inflammatory effects on this process via reinvigoration of pro-inflammatory cytokines and increased antioxidant protection. Furthermore, both physical and mental effects of exercise such as anti-stress and happiness contribute to the entire wellbeing hence making one immune against aged associated diseases.

Besides lifestyle modifications, pharmacological agents aimed at modulating selective inflammatory and oxidative pathways are potential candidates that may assist in slowing down aging and longevity. Compounds such as resveratrol, curcumin, and polyphenols we display excellent antioxidative and anti-inflammatory power bearing a probable medical potential in aging related chronic diseases.

Additionally, contemporary researches show that intermittent-fasting and calorie restriction modulate the inflammatory responses and increase cellular stress resistance strengthening longevity in various organisms e.g from yeast to mammalian physiology.

The convergence of scientific findings underscores the critical importance of addressing inflammation and oxidative stress in the pursuit of longevity and optimal health. By embracing lifestyle modifications, dietary interventions, and pharmacological strategies, individuals can potentially forestall age-related decline and pave the way towards a vibrant and fulfilling life.

- **Anti-Inflammatory Agents: From Natural Compounds to Pharmaceutical Interventions**

The investigation of anti-inflammatory agents is a vital line, which could be pathway to treatment of chronic inflammation and age-related pathologies. This investigation straddles a broad continuum starting from the natural compounds coming out of plants to an advanced area on pharmacology ameliorated by medical treatment science.

Finding new, breakthrough anti-inflammatory agents outside the scientific labs is impossible as polyphenols – omnipresent in fruits, legumes, and herbs – surface as worthy competitors to artificial drugs. Their efficacy stems from a multifaceted approach: Antioxidant properties, inhibition of pro-inflammatory enzymes and modification of the immune system's functioning. The endogenous richness in polyphenols from which plant-based origin not only delineates their potency as therapeutic analogs but also reflects the abstract of holistic health advancement.

On the other hand, the physicians' pharmaceutical armamentarium of interventions presents a NSAIDs and cytokine-targeted therapies. NSAIDs, while widely used for their potent anti-inflammatory effects, come tethered to a caveat: adverse effects that may include side gastrointestinal problems, varying from disturbances to cardiovascular complication. This paradox throws light on the importance of safer and more effective alternatives as a compromise in this environment, where the answer potentially lies.

The story of discovery and convergence between natural substance entities and innovative pharmaceuticals unfolds as a timeline before reducing the effects of any inflammation. With the growing evidence provided by research that deepens our comprehension of inflammatory pathways and details on age-related inflammation, it is possible to integrate interpretation of the modes in which natural compounds function and how pharmaceutical treatments should be initiated with promising results – transformation outcomes.

In fact, the survey of anti-inflammatory compounds crosses off scientific disciplinary partition walls grafting phytochemical knowledge with pharmacological information and a clinical approach. Inside this discovery landscape lies the opportunity to remold new paradigms of health-care, a time where inflammation enshrouds aging as an unavoidable sign yet now becomes another part merited for prevention and reinstitution for optimal functioning and wellness.

- ## Antioxidant Strategies: Harnessing the Power of Nutraceuticals and Lifestyle Interventions

In an active pursuit of increasing lifespan and general positive health, antioxidant strategies serve as a crucial focal point. This tactic is revealing the utility of antioxidants in the domain of nutraceuticals and lifestyle interventions, specifically addressing aging-linked oxidative stress implication to complications development.

Antioxidants are like defenders, since they neutralize the free radicals—the molecules disrupting cell structures. Among them vitamins C and E, glutathione as well as coenzyme Q10 may be mentioned. Meaning that antioxidants help condemn these radicals by 'donating' electrons to them. Additionally, these substances support the body' endogenic antioxidant defense system, strengthening cells against oxidative stress.

The other aspect in these defensive strategies is nutraceuticals that comprise of antioxidants. Vitamin C is present in high amounts of all varieties of citrus fruits and most leafy vegetables which scavenges free radicals but regenerates the action of vitamin E hence accentuating its protective effects. It works synergistically with vitamin C to prevent intracellular oxidative stress, wherein it attacks the nucleus of the cell in an attempt to destroy it. Vitamin E is widely present as nuts and seeds while vegetable oils do have this particular nutrient. Made in the body from amino acid precursors glutathione is a master antioxidant, coordinating all of nature's free radicals and toxic molecules to safely detoxify them. The function of organ meats and oily fish is not only the prevention oxidative stress, but also assists mitochondria's internal apparatus which leads to cellular energy production.

However, the complementary role of lifestyle modifications, such as changes in a person's diet and way of life, cannot be overstated while talking about the alleviation of oxidative stress and facilitation of longevity. Regular exercise increases antioxidant enzyme activity, stimulates mitochondrial function, and reduces inflammation- it all boils down to preventing oxidative damage through consumption of supplements that maintain the following cells. These include dietary changes that focus mainly at antioxidant-rich foods, including berries, leafy greens and nuts providing the body with a continuous source of anti-oxidants which strengthens its defense systems. Additionally, stress management methodologies such as mindfulness meditation and deep breathing workouts allow to mitigate the negative influence of chronic stress over cellular integrity thus providing an opportunity for decreasing oxidative burden.

The integration of antioxidant strategies—both through nutraceutical interventions and lifestyle modifications—represents a holistic approach to fortifying cellular resilience, mitigating oxidative stress, and fostering longevity. By embracing these strategies, individuals can empower themselves to navigate the challenges of aging and disease with vigor and vitality.

Overall, inflammation and oxidative stress-based antiaging can be concluded into a prominent paradigm of improving life length and health span. So, by disentangling the highly orchestrated molecular machineries that shape inflammation and oxidative stress damage; scientists would aim at bringing in new therapeutic interventions as well as lifestyle practices to age cells back without depriving them of their physiological status. Herein, we explore the science that underlies human longevity and discuss how to use this knowledge regarding inflammation, oxidative stress, senescence-related mechanisms and other associated health concerns to our advantage in navigating the process of aging.

5.4. Clinical Considerations and Emerging Research on Metformin for Longevity

In recent years, Metformin has emerged as a promising candidate for extending longevity and promoting healthy aging. Originally developed as a frontline treatment for type 2 diabetes, Metformin's potential to influence metabolic and cellular processes associated with aging has garnered significant attention from researchers and healthcare practitioners alike. In this section, we explore the clinical considerations and the latest findings from emerging research on Metformin's role in promoting longevity and enhancing overall health.

- ### Metformin: A Diabetes Medication with Longevity Benefits

Metformin is one of the key medications in the fight against type 2 diabetes and it not only shows up as the pivot in glycemic control but also shows an inspiring side of longevity. Its polyvalent mechanism induces revolutionary responses in metabolic pathways being a new era for therapeutic opportunities beyond glucose control.

At the center of Metformin's efficacy is the modulation of AMP-activated protein kinase (AMPK), a critical central regulator mediating cellular energy balance. Activation of AMPK by Metformin initiates a series of downstream events which ultimately seeks to remedy metabolic imbalance. Metformin enhances glucose uptake in peripheral tissues thereby boosting insulin sensitivity and leading to better utilization of circulating glucose. In addition, its suppression of liver gluconeogenesis prevents the hyperglycemia caused by glucose overproduction in the liver which is a hallmark of DGL.

The action of metformin goes beyond glucose metabolism and incorporates lipid metabolism. By increasing fatty acid oxidation, it controls lipid accumulation and prevents the maladaptive outcomes of dyslipidemia that are common in diabetic patients. This broad modulation of metabolic pathways prepares a body for better glycemic regulation and prevents the detrimental effects of metabolic disarrangement.

Interestingly, the preventative effects of Metformin are not limited to diabetes management. Novel evidence hints on the relationship between Metformin and longevity, opening up a new window of research regarding its anti-aging attributes. Metformin extends longevity and delays age-related pathologies; experimental models and epidemiological studies have revealed tantalizingly promising glimpses of Metformin's transformative capacity towards aging well.

Metformin stands as a beacon of hope in the management of type 2 diabetes, underpinned by its multifaceted modulation of metabolic pathways. Its burgeoning role in the realm of longevity underscores its significance beyond glycemic control, paving the way for a paradigm shift in our approach to chronic disease management and healthy aging.

- **Effects on Aging Processes**

Becoming a forte of antidiabetic, Metformin extends beyond its prime pharmacological role to demonstrate promising effects upon aging processes and age-associated disorders. Despite scrutiny through a vast body of preclinical studies scrutinizing nematodes, fruit flies, and rodents, Metformin transpires as a unique agent that, in its capacity to prolong life and prevent age-related syndromes such as cardiovascular complications, Alzheimer's disease, and cancer.

At the heart of metformin's prowess is its unique ability to regulate cellular pathways that contribute to metabolism, inflammation, and oxidative stress hence aiding in the aging process. Metformin entwines with these labyrinthine pathways, creating a choir of effects that harmonizes with the very existence of longevity and life-force.

Metformin should be ranked among the top areas through which this medicine flexes its therapeutic muscles and influence the process of metabolism. Through metabolic fine-tuning, Metformin does more than just attenuate glucose dysregulation; this drug also sets a series of events that result in better energy consumption and enhanced cellular wellbeing: one of the most distinctive characteristics of youth.

Moreover, Metformin makes its appearance as a stern antagonist in the confrontation with raging pro-inflammatory surge that comes along with aging. Starting the age-related inflammation at bay by controlling its inflammatory patterns, Metformin stands as a sizeable wall against age inflammation that creates an atmosphere that favors cell neoplasms, Metformin does not favor a cell neoplasms ambiance; in other words, the explanation holds true in the statement that by the containing the cascading

After Metformin, oxidative stress, the bother of aging itself has met its match, its nemesis and its downfall. Being an antioxidant, Metformin is a pioneer in the fight against oxidative ravages that drive the aging pathways of various organisms. With scavenging free radicals, enhancing endogenous antioxidant potency erects a barrier, a standing shield for cellular sturdiness and resilience, rolling back the incipient effects of oxidative stress on ageing organ.

Metformin transcends its antidiabetic confines to emerge as a beacon of hope in the realm of aging research. By modulating cellular signaling pathways implicated in metabolism, inflammation, and oxidative stress, Metformin unveils a multifaceted approach towards promoting longevity and combating age-related ailments, thereby offering a glimmer of promise in the quest for eternal youthfulness.

- **<u>Clinical Evidence in Human Studies</u>**

Clinical evidence in human studies is a vital link between emerging hopeful preclinical data and everyday therapeutic use that may be applied in clinical practice. Regarding Metformin, a drug that is often used to manage diabetes, scientists have been looking at its possible use a longevity promoting agent, especially among elderly group of individuals. Metformin as a broad drug across various areas of application beyond glycemic control can be understood only with the depth of understanding of clinical evidence.

The observational studies form the beginning of Metformin's evaluation as age-outcomes. These are observational studies where the participants are observed for duration to determine the correlations between Metformin use and all health parameters. For example, a seminal study published in Journal of the American Geriatrics Society investigated older adults with type 2 diabetes and revealed that Metformin users have an increased rate of all-cause mortality and a reduced incidence of age-associated diseases compared to non-Metformin users. Such results provide suggestive and profound perspectives on effects of Metformin beyond glycemic control in aged populations.

Nevertheless, observational studies are limited by the possibility of confounding factors which can lead to confounding bias. Thus, robust clinical trials give support to the proof of causality and effectiveness of Metformin for longevity promotion. In this context, the Targeting Aging with Metformin (TAME) trial emanates as a pioneering initiative. This long-running trial seeks to measure the effectiveness of preventing the advent of age-related diseases and lengthening healthspan in non-diabetics by administering Metformin.

The design of the TAME trial outlines a kind of holistic approach to the assessment of Metformin's geroprotective potential. Through investigation of the sum of the composite outcome, cardiovascular events, cancer incidence, cognitive decline and mortality, the trial tackles the complex nature of aging-related health outcomes. This holistic assessment allows the researchers to reflect the wide range of the effects Metformin has on humans' life and longevity.

Furthermore, using randomized controlled trials, the TAME trial involves rigorous methodology and minimizes bias within the study. By balancing confounding variables, randomization promotes the relevance of the results. Furthermore, longitudinal follow-up enables researchers to calculate the long-term effects of Metformin on aging-related outcomes.

Past the TAME trial, other clinical studies help the evidence of Metformin as a geroprotective agent. These researches review different elements of Metformin's pharmacodynamics, an ideal dose, and duration of its use, as well as its possible combination with other medications. By conducting a systematic review and meta-analysis of previous literature, researchers will aggregate findings emanating from different studies to draw more reliable conclusions regarding Metformin's effectiveness and safety profile.

Clinical evidences from human studies have a valuable role in clarifying Metformin's potential for use as a life-extending intervention. Ranging from observational studies that emphasize relationships between Metformin use and better health outcomes to clinical trials as TAME on a large scale, researchers are developing knowledge about the role of Metformin in normal aging. They integrate numerous methodologies and systematically evaluation them, which allows clinical practice and health policy to make informed decisions.

- ## Safety and Considerations for Long-Term Use

For drugs like Metformin, which have a lifelong use, safety is one of the most critical aspects due to its general prescription. Although Metformin has been recognized as one of the cornerstones in the treatment of type-2 diabetes, due to its safety and efficacy in management, it is essential to understand the possible limitations, as well as unwanted actions as a possible consequence of prolonged use of Metformin.

For many years, metformin, which is a biguanide derivative, has remained the hallmark of type 2 diabetes management. Its main mechanism underlies lowing of hepatic glucose production and improving of peripheral tissue's sensitivity to insulin. Nonetheless Metformin, similarly to any medicine, is not absolutely free of side effects and risks hence presupposes constant observation and risk-benefit analysis during the course of long-term usage.

However, gastrointestinal disturbances are one of the most prevalent sources of adverse results that can be observed in connection with Metformin. This usually leads to symptoms that are common to the patients like diarrhea, nausea, and abdominal discomforts; this is particularly realized when therapy begins or when dosages are increased. These side effects can add some kind of nuisance and causing in non-compliance of medicinal dosage or even the withdrawal of medication use. Physicians need to inform the patients regarding the associated adverse effects of such diversion effects and prescribe the mitigation strategies in terms of taking Metformin with meals or incorporating the extended-release versions to lessen the impact.

Other than gastrointestinal problems, Metformin is linked with adverse side effects that could be very serious and include lactic acidosis. The disease is mainly a metabolic complication associated with the lactic acidosis that leads to the elevated level of lactate in the blood that, in turn, causes both systemic acidosis. The risk of lactic acidosis, however, remains low even though the absolute risk is higher in individuals who already have predisposing factors like renal impaction, hepatic dysfunction, or conditions that are closely associated with tissue hypoxia. Therefore, proper screening and monitoring of renal function would be critical before initiating Metformin therapy, as well as at subsequent intervals when dealing with the vulnerable population.

Additionally, clinicians should be careful prescribing Metformin to the elder population or patients with large numbers of comorbidities since they are likely to have unfavorable reactions and need tight supervision. Precise treatment protocols that are tailored according to the various characteristics of the patients and risk factors are essential for ensuring the best treatment outcomes with minimal risks.

Aside from adverse effect monitoring, the long-term effects of Metformin treatment on the organ systems, are also issues that need to be considered by clinicians. Although there is extensive clinical evidence supports that Metformin is tolerated well over long-term exposure, research is required to evaluate the association with cardiovascular recovery, bone metabolism, and cancer risk. Some studies have shown that Metformin use may have cardio protection benefits while others have toned a note of caution on its adverse effects on vitamin B12 levels and bone health. It is therefore recommended that clinicians continuously monitor new evidence in relation to Metformin and continuously update recommendations which should be implemented into clinical practice to ensure best use of Metformin.

Although Metformin is an essential component of the treatment for people with type 2 diabetes, physicians should be cautious and watch for the side effects and long-term impacts of this drug. Thinking through patient risk factors, adverse effects, and current available research, practitioners can ensure that Metformin therapy treated diabetes and other metabolic conditions in an optimum manner.

In conclusion, Metformin has emerged as a promising candidate for use as an anti-aging agent. Its multipronged mechanisms of action, coupled with its good safety profile and a wealth of preclinical and clinical data, make a tantalizing geroprotective agent. With research revealing the drug's effects on aging processes and age-related diseases, the ongoing endeavor to optimize the dose regimens, identify responder phenotypes, and explore the combination therapies leaves hope for using the drug's full potential in enhancing longevity and health outcomes among the heterogenous population.

CHAPTER 6
UNDERSTANDING ACARBOSE

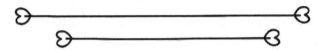

6.1.   Mechanism of Action: Slowing Carbohydrate Breakdown and Reducing Glucose Spikes

T he study of the mechanisms of action, within the fields of pharmacology and medical science, is critical for the implementation of successful treatment plans. From all these mechanisms, the pathway through which the rate of carbohydrates and glucose spikes are reduced is one of the most important ones, especially when it comes to the management of conditions such as diabetes mellitus and metabolic disorders. This article discusses the complex course of this mechanism, clarifying its physiological bases and clinical connotations.

- **Carbohydrate Metabolism: A Fundamental Process**

Under the human nutrition, carbohydrates are seen as the central pillars because of their role as the fundamental source of energy necessary for sustaining the body physiological processes. The drinking of various carbohydrate-containing foodstuffs such as cereals, fruits, vegetables etc., mark the beginning of the complex metabolism. With the digestion, theses carbohydrates experience a series of complicated enzymatic reactions that result in the formation of glucose, the main energy source comprised to cells' energy cycles.

In the context of the intestinal tract, carbohydrates interact with a wide range of enzymes that catalyze for their breakage into simple sugars. The enzyme maltase splits the polysaccharides, which are secreted by the salivary glands and the pancreas gland, to monosaccharides like maltose and sucrose. Following these, the enzymes such as maltase and sucrase break down these disaccharides into glucose in more specific monosaccharide components, most of which are glucose.

At the same time, glucose occupies the highest position in the hierarchy of carbohydrate break down and has ultimate significance for cellular energetics. After being taken up by the blood plasma, glucose acts as an immediate substrate for tissues and organs, and their continual functioning is due to successful metabolism. Regulation of proper amount of blood glucose is a challenge that only an orchestra of hormones, especially the insulin and the glucan, can achieve.

Insulin, produced and released by pancreatic β-cells as part of the anabolism process upon seeing an increase in glucose level in the blood stream, enables the uptake of glucose by different tissues such as muscle, adipose tissue, and the liver. Following the binding of insulin to its receptors, GLUT proteins are translocated to the cell membrane and serve as the channels through which glucose enters the cytoplasm itself. Herein is the basis for glucose uptake as glucose undergoes glycolysis—a metabolic chain of events giving ATP, considered the energy currency.

On the other hand, in the instances of vigorous fasting or blood low glucose levels, the pancreas gives out glucagon, which controls mobilization of glycogen from hepatic sources. The other pathway the glycogenolysis breaks down glycogen to glucose-6-phosphate which provides immediate glucose for tissues having energy demands. Additionally, in long-term fasting state or under condition of strenuous exercise where glucose is needed, gluconeogenesis is kicked into gear—a process whereby these non-carbohydrate precursors such as amino acids and glycerol are converted into glucose by the liver and kidneys.

On the other hand, disturbances originating from carbohydrate metabolism can predispose to disorders of metabolism particularly diabetes mellitus. Type 1 diabetes develops as a result of the destruction of pancreatic beta cells due to autoimmunity, which leads to an insulin deficiency and an uncontrolled high blood sugar level. On the other hand, type 2 diabetes results from insulin resistance, a malaise where target organs have a reduced response to insulin signaling and hence impaired uptake and utilization of glucose. The subsequent hyperglycemia leads to the disseminated complications known as cardiovascular disease, neuropathy, and nephropathy revealing the importance of carbohydrate homeostasis.

In addition, imbalance in carbohydrate metabolism is much wider than diabetes, involving metabolic syndrome, obesity, and dyslipidemia. Not only do these pathologies affect metabolic health but they also predispose patients to an increased cardiovascular morbidity and mortality.

Thus, carbohydrate metabolism is one of the primary physiological processes in cells that ensure the cellular energetics and metabolic homeostasis persistence. Any step of carbohydrate metabolism, such as enzymatic decomposition in the gastrointestinal tract, and the intricate sequential scheme of hormonal regulation, highlights the sophisticated coordination of biochemical pathways. Nevertheless, disturbances in carbohydrate metabolism may trigger a chain of metabolic consequences in this context the critical need to keep glucose homeostasis in order to ensure optimal health conditions is stressed.

- <u>Acarbose: Unveiling its Mode of Action</u>

A potent and reliable drug for diabetes management is acarbose, considered the best friend to manage type 2 diabetes mellitus. What comes to perfection is the intricate modulation of carbohydrate metabolism through a unique mode of action where the drug influences the following actions in sequential order. acarbose can be seen as an alpha-glucosidase inhibitor that works in tine gastrointestinal repository whereby it has the control over the enzymes that are responsible for the digests along with that part of the carbohydrate where they are absorbed.

The beginning of acarbose's action path is identified with an artificial postponement of carbohydrate degradation due to its strategic intrusion into complex processes of carbohydrate breakdown. When they are ingested, carbohydrates from diet in turn are met with the digestive capacities of alpha-glucosidase enzymes in the brush border of the small intestine. These enzymes serve as important, namely maltase, sucrase, and glucoamylase, as they break such complex carbohydrates to other simple glucose molecules that may be absorbed into blood for any purpose. From all this, we see the essence of acarbose's power

Acarbose, a pseudo-tetrasaccharide that is obtained from bacterial fermentation work as a powerful inhibitor of alpha-glucosidase enzymes through the inhibition of the production of glucose produced form non-carbohydrate substances. It does so by practically competitive inhibiting these enzymes' active sites, leading to prevention of hydrolysis of complex carbohydrates into absorbable glucose molecules. As a result, digestion and absorption of carbohydrates to a great extent are being significantly delayed and weakened.

Every wagon of the train echoes with the reverberations of acarbose which are due to the inhibitory effects that prolong postprandial spikes of blood glucose in diabetes. Composed of this action, depicted above as an impediment to carbohydrate digestion and absorption, acarbose orchestrates a more gradual and effaced release of glucose into the bloodstream subsequent to meals. This level of attenuation of type 2 diabetes mellitus postprandial hyperglycemia functions as the foundation of the integrated management of type 2 diabetes mellitus.

Other physiological changes that acarbose induces but are not directly related to carbohydrate metabolism may synergize with the immediate effects to improve efficacy The delayed carbohydrate absorption allows for a subtle calibration of insulin secretion such that the system is protected from the dramatic oscillations in glucose levels which would cause insulin to be released to an outrageous degree. This subtle dialectic finely balancing the action of acarbose, glucose, and insulin signals for a subtler beat in the intricate metabolic architecture.

Moreover, acarbose potency touches not only on blood sugar control but also on acarbose's lipid metabolism effects as mentioned before. Acarbose blunts the influx of glucose into the bloodstream and thus attenuates the lipogenic response following the release of insulin; this coupled with the fact that insulin drives the synthesis of triglycerides in adipose tissue means that the effect of acarbose on the lipogenic pathway is to attenuate the production and accum The dual action on carbohydrate and lipid metabolism also highlights some of the wide-ranging advantages of acarbose in alleviating the cardiovascular risk profile account of diabetic patients.

Beyond the effectiveness of acarbose within its efficacy, in a clinical domain, the potential therapeutic use of acarbose is embedded in action with other antidiabetic agents. In combination therapy that balances the actions on insulin sensitizers, sulfonylureas and the incretin-based therapies, acarbose offers great versatility in the personalized management of diabetes to a wide range of practitioners, thus helping to minimize the impact of the disease on both patients and practitioners.

- **Slowing Carbohydrate Breakdown: The Alpha-Glucosidase Inhibition**

In the pharmacology and the cycle of metabolism acarbose's function of operation is enshrined in its ability to control the carbohydrates metabolic rates by targeting the alpha-glucosidase enzymes in the intestine's brush border. This mechanism is a pivotal structure enacting in the control of various metabolic disorders primarily type 2 diabetes mellitus.

Basically, alpha-glucosidase enzymatic activity performs hydrolysis of the rather complicated carbohydrates into both monosaccharides, in particular, glucose, that is responsible for the absorption of the sugar into the blood. In contrast, acarbose, an active alpha-glucosidase inhibitor, demonstrates its curative power by the begone of these important enzymes, thus stifling their catalytic activity.

The competitive inhibition which acarbose's operation entails; disrupts the enzymatic breakdown of polysaccharides, preventing the conversion of complex carbohydrates into glucose units that the body can absorb. As a result, the movement of glucose is significantly inhibited, which aims to transmit reactive hyperglycemia, a distinctive feature of diabetes mellitus.

The complexities of the action mechanism of acarbose refers, on the one hand, to particularity towards alpha-glucosidase type enzymes, sparing other digestive enzymes from the inhibitory effect of the substance. By the intervention directed specifically, you can modulate the carbohydrate digestion process selectively, preserving the overall structural integrity of the above digestive function.

In addition acarbose hinders carbohydrate breakdown and this implies that following meals blood sugar levels do not increase abruptly but gradually and steadily which is a way of averting the deleterious impacts eglomise of blood sugar levels.

Clinically, acarbose has a therapeutic utility, which harkens beyond glycemic control, but also includes anti- metabolic-syndrome pharmacology and obesity management. Its effectiveness in reducing hyperglycemia that follows meals makes the drug an excellent ancillary management agent alongside lifestyle changes and other pharmacological agents in the comprehensive treatment of metabolic disorders.

In brief, the deep modulation of metabolism of sugar through enzyme inhibitions uses acarbose as it discovered and an important source of fighting metabolic disorders.

- **Reducing Glucose Spikes: Mitigating Postprandial Hyperglycemia**

Postprandial hyperglycemia is a food-induced condition characterized by high serum glucose levels after eating and it poses a major challenge especially to those with defective carbohydrate metabolism, especially diabetics. While transient fasting hyperglycemia has short-term consequences, repercussions such as cardiovascular disease or neuropathy can persist into the long-term. One pharmacological agent that can address this challenge is acarbose, which is famous for its capabilities of dealing with postprandial hyperglycemia by modulation of carbohydrate digestion.

Acarbose functions through inhibition of the rapid digestion of complex carbohydrates into simple sugars from the digestive tract. Acarbose, instead, functions by restricting the operation of the enzymes α-glucosidase that are necessary in transforming the complex carbohydrates into glucose that can be absorbed. This reduces carbohydrate absorption rate which equals to slow release of glucose to the blood, leading to the blunted blood glucose post meal rise in patient with Type 2 diabetes.

The action mechanism of acarbose is in line with the basic principle of glycemic control, implying managing the blood glucose levels to remain within a minute physiological range. Acarbose slower absorption of glucose into the bloodstream after meals, which, in turn, increases the patients' glycemic stability, as well as decreases risks of hyperglycemic episodes occurrence, and thus minimizes the risk of late complications of the conduction.

Additionally, acarbose provides an adjoined modality of diabetes treatment along with the lifestyle changes and other drug approaches that help to improve blood glucose control. It has been studied clinically and shown to be effective in reducing postprandial hyperglycemia and therefore, it serves as the main deal of therapy in the treatment of diabetes and other metabolic disorders.

It can be concluded that metalloenzyme inhibitor acarbose can be an efficient therapeutic agent if administered to patients with impaired carbohydrates metabolism as regular treatment for postprandial hyperglycemia reduction and prevention of diabetes-related complications. Through the modular abilities of carbohydrate digestion, acarbose can be regarded as one of the pharmacological approaches that provide glycemic control and also maintain optimal therapeutic outcomes among diabetic patients.

- **Clinical Implications and Therapeutic Considerations**

Acarbose is a medicine used for treatment conditions related to diabetes mellitus and other metabolic disorders, mainly altering carbohydrate metabolism and reducing PPMGs. This feature is also immensely important from a therapeutic perspective in the case of diabetes, particularly in terms of the enhanced ability to reach optimized glycemic and allay the risk of diabetic complications.

Acarbose is frequently used as a biological component that is incorporated in clinical practices as an important part of a comprehensive diabetes care plan among lifestyle adjustments and other pharmacological treatment arsenal like insulin and oral hypoglycemic medicines. A salient feature of the disease process is that even though hyperglycemia is the primary metabolic imbalance, various pathophysiological developments, such as α-cell ultrastructural alterations , could cause distinct and irregular responses on glycemic control of diabetes patients.

Acarbose works as an inhibitor of alpha-glucosidase enzymes located in the small intestine, which leads to the constraint of the digestion and absorption of complicated sugars. In result, the postprandial spike in glucose concentration is reduced resulting in relatively uniformed and consistent patterns of glycemic response across the day. This mechanism is quite useful in type 2 diabetic patients, in whom PP hyperglycemia has a heavy role on the glycemic management as well as vascular complication.

In addition, the use of acarbose can lower the possibility of hypoglycemia, a side effect which frequently appears when using other medicines designed for diabetes treatment such as insulin and sulfonylureas. By virtue of its extraordinary way of action, it primarily affects the postprandial stages of glucose without substantially changing the fasting concentrations of glucose; thus, its efficacy in maintaining glycemia ranges between moderate attempts of breaking through decreases or increases.

When deciding to implant acarbose in an individual's treatment routine, there are several things to be taken into consideration by clinicians, such as blood glucose goals, renal function, gastrointestinal developments as well as any possible medication interactions. It is essential to promote close monitoring and periodic review of the glycemic parameters to ensure the best clinical response with minimum aspiration

Acarbose represents a valuable therapeutic option in the management of diabetes mellitus, offering a targeted approach to glycemic control and reducing the risk of diabetic complications. Its integration into comprehensive treatment plans underscores the importance of personalized care in achieving optimal clinical outcomes for patients with diabetes and related metabolic disorders.

The inhibition of carbohydrate breakdown and the suppression of glucose spikes by the same mechanism of action serves as a milestone in the treatment of diabetes mellitus and well as metabolic disorders, already represented by acarbose and like drugs. Acarbose inhibits alpha -glucosidase enzymes in a highly specific manner and controls postprandial carbohydrate metabolism, leading to glycemic normalization and amelioration of the after-meal hyperglycemia mediated complications. Through their elucidation of these complex interactions between the pharmacological measures and physiological processes, clinicians and researchers can continue to refine treatment modalities and increase favorable treatment outcomes in the field of metabolic health.

6.2.   Influence on Glycation and Oxidative Stress: Implications for Aging Processes

Glycation and oxidative stress represent two interconnected processes that play pivotal roles in the aging of biological systems. Understanding their influence and implications is essential for elucidating the mechanisms underlying aging processes and developing interventions aimed at promoting longevity and vitality.

- **<u>Glycation: The Molecular Link to Aging</u>**

The singular protein event, called the glycation, which occurs between sugars and biomolecules as we age, interprets the ambiguity of action which is the flux of time. Glycation is the non-enzymatic bonding of sugars, especially glucose, to proteins, lipids, or nucleic acids to form advanced glycation end products (AGEs). This phenomenon follows an inherent part of physiological metabolism and promotes acceleration under hyperglycemia and over-heightened oxidative stress environment.

Cellular and tissue organisms' homeostasis through AGEs, the products of glycation, imply significant deeds. They demonstrate an innate tendency to amass in different tissues and organs through the tides, necessitating structural and functional adaptation. These variations that epitomize age-related disease pathologies uncover the complex dance between glycation and aging.

The deleterious effects of glycation span the breadth of organismal realms. Notably, glycation seems to interfere with the conformational integrity of proteins, hinder enzymatic function, and thus hamper many of the signaling events in cells that rely on molecular recognition. On the other hand, lipid glycation can lead to the first step of oxidative stress, facilitate lipid peroxidation, and create a favorable environment for atherosclerosis and neurodegeneration. In addition, there is evidence nucleic acid glycation may lead to DNA damage due to the damaging effects of glycation products on the integrity of the genomic structure and lead to the start of mutagenic cascades.

The discovery of the broad ramifications of glycation is also tantalizing in terms of potential for medical intervention to manage age-related disorders. Since research has been able to guide at the molecular level to describe glycation decrypts, there can be a solution can be able to mitigate its adverse downfalls. Such concerted efforts at the elucidation of glycation on the subsequent stages are to shed new light on the mechanisms of healthspan extension and the alleviation of the age-related morbidity burden.

- **The Impact of Glycation on Aging**

Glycation is one of the main processes in aging, occurring in an advanced glycation end product (AGE), arising when sugars react with proteins, lipids, and nucleic acids. It is huge and multifaceted, affecting a number of biomolecules and physiological functions depending on the aging process.

In glycation, proteins are modified in size, shape, and function. These changes give rise to reduction in the flexibility and changes in interaction with other molecules. As a result, functioning of enzymes, receptors, and structural proteins is impaired. This structural alteration affects their physiological capacity to function, thus directly contributing to the age related loss in the function of the tissue and of the organs.

In addition, the accumulation of AGE leads to increasing inflammation and oxidative stress, intensifying tissue injury and contributing to the development of age-related conditions such as diabetes, heart diseases, and neurodegenerative diseases. Chronic inflammation and oxidative stress building a hostile environment for cells and tissues including their degeneration and their impairment to the best functions.

One of the other effects of glycation is the connection of proteins which undermines the tissue elasticity. This dynamic leads to the hardening of blood vessels, skin, and connective tissues that are typical of the ageing process. Age-related stiffening of these structures has both mechanical and functional implications as they render the normal functioning of the structures impossible, causing a number of age-related complications.

Overall, glycation plays an important role in the process of aging through the changes of biomolecular structure and function, oxidative stress and tissue elasticity. The understanding of the cellular and molecular mechanisms involved in the glycation process is essential for the design of interventions to prevent or manage the adverse outcomes of the glycation process and promote a successful aging process.

- **Oxidative Stress: The Role of Reactive Oxygen Species**

Oxidative stress is one of the most integral concepts in the description of balance within biological systems. In essence, the fundamental cause of oxidative stress is the relative dominance of reactive oxygen species (ROS) over the antioxidant defense mechanisms of body. These ROS occurring in cells as superoxide radicals, hydrogen peroxide, hydroxyl radicals, among other free radicals arise from cellular metabolic activity and external factors such as radiation and pollutants.

Within the intricacies of cellular biology, ROS play dual roles: first, as important signaling molecules which play a crucial role in regulating a wide range of physiological functions and second, major sources of cellular injury when they get over accumulated. Basic processes of oxidative stress rely on ROS promoted oxidation of essential biomolecules such as proteins, lipids, and

DNA. It is following oxidative alterations that can lead to disruption of cellular structures, enzyme inhibition, and even cellular mutations that can affect integrity and activity of cells.

More importantly, the effects of oxidative stress do not remain limited to cellular failure, but also predispose to a variety of diseases in pathogenesis e.g. cancer, neurodegenerative disorders, and cardiovascular diseases. In fact, the harmful properties of oxidants reinforce the importance of a well-balanced ROS production and antioxidant defense mechanisms.

As oxidative stress is characterized by its multi-layered nature, it is apparent that any interventions that target regulation of the levels of reactive oxygen species ROS show great potential in treatment. In particular, dietary antioxidants, life adjustments, and medication therapies are promising sources for the reduction of the harmful effects of oxidative stress and the maintenance of general health and quality of life.

With a deeper and broader understanding of ROS kinetics and antioxidant systems, scientists and physicians are trying to untangle the mysteries of oxidative stress bringing about groundbreaking therapeutic options.

- ## **The Impact of Oxidative Stress on Aging**

Oxidative stress emerges as a critical link to the complex structure of aging biology and the initiating point of a cascade of cellular events giving shape to the aging phenotype. Basically, oxidative stress results from the imbalance of production and the protective response by antioxidant mechanisms of reactive oxygen species (ROS) systems. The accumulation of ROS, as this phenomenon is described, initiates a set of molecular responses that alter considerably the physiology of the cells and facilitate the aging of the organism.

The oxidative stress is associated with the harmful and damaging properties against the cellular components such as lipids, proteins as well as DNA. There are three types of ROS- mediated lipid peroxidation, protein oxidation and DNA damage then ROS have the function of hallmarks of oxidative stress- mediated cellular dysfunction. As a result, such molecular offenses impair cellular homeostasis and interfere with vital cellular processes, paving the way for cellular senescence, apoptosis, and genomic instability.

Of significant interest is the susceptibility of mitochondria to oxidative injury due to its dual character as both the beginning and end of ROS. Crucial organelles in the form of mitochondria that is responsible for regulating energy production and cellular metabolism becomes vulnerable to potential oxidative insults and rendering their functionality. Therefore, a consequence of this is mitochondrial disorder, which leads to increased production of ROS, thus incessantly triggering a circle of oxidative stress.

Briefly, oxidative stress appears as a central factor governing this process, operating through a multitude of molecular pathways affecting the stability and paramount functions of every living cell. The ability to unravel the complex overlay between ROS and cell physiology may lead to illuminating approaches to the apt response to oxidative stress and boosting healthy human lives.

- **Implications for Aging Processes**

The processes of aging are strictly conjugated with the glycation and oxidative stress – two primary mechanisms that appear to have a great impact on the onset and development of age-related diseases. AGEs are formed from the glycations non-enzymatic response between sugars and proteins. These AGEs are over time produced and lead to harmful impact on the cellular functions and tissues.

In addition to glycation, oxidative stress, the excess overbalance between free radicals and antioxidants in the body contributes to more severe damage to cells and faster development of the aging processes. The cumulative effect of chronic accumulation of AGEs and resultant oxidative damage is involved in a number of other age-related pathologies, including diabetes, cardiovascular diseases, Alzheimer's disease, and osteoporosis.

Additionally, the damage that glycation and oxidative stress cause affects the structure and function that changes in aging skin. These changes present themselves with sagginess, loss of elasticity, poor wound healing, reflecting the molecular and cellular abnormalities.

The pivotal importance of glycation and oxidative stress in the process of aging and the possibility of intervening in these processes are quite promising paths that might lead to healthy aging and increased lifespan. Antiglycation measures for the prevention of glycation would include a reduction of dietary glucose intake and the employment of pharmacological interventions that have the potential to limit AGE formation. In a similar vein supporting antioxidant defenses with lifestyle modifications and supplementation may address oxidative stress and blunt its negative effects on aging tissues.

In conclusion, such understanding of glycation and oxidative stress allows one to see the mechanism marking processes of aging and facilitates the development of such strategies that will ensure healthspan enrichment and longevity promotion.

- ### <u>Therapeutic Approaches to Target Glycation and Oxidative Stress</u>

The desire to improve the adverse effects of glycation and oxidative stress on aging has spurred different treatment approaches which include; diet modifications, antioxidant supplements and drug intervention. These strategies are aimed at counteracting the negative effects of the advanced glycation end-products and reactive oxygen species accumulation – significant components of the aging process.

Within the framework of therapeutics, dietary changes serve as a basis. The inclusion of nutrient-dense foods containing high antioxidant and low sugars is an effective approach in attenuating glycation and oxidative stress. At the same time, supplementation with antioxidants like ascorbic acid, tocopherols, and polyphenols provides specific protection against ROS-induced damage, strengthening cellular resistance and enhancing life.

Additionally, some compounds have drawn interest with regard to antiglycation effects. Primarily, carnosine – a natural dipeptide, and pyridoxamine – a form of vitamin B6, have extremely potent anti-glycation properties, preventing AGEs and thus, preventing further downstream pathological profiles.

Pharmacological intervention that is meant to intercept the glycation and oxidative stress pathways constitutes another area in therapeutic innovation. Acting as selective regulators of enzymatic processes associated with glycation in addition to strengthening endogenous antioxidant defense mechanisms these agents are potentially effective in preventing the age-related degeneration as well as extending the period of health.

These therapeutic modalities provide a holistic approach to combat glycation, oxidative stress, among others, which form the foundation for the pursuit of viable anti-aging strategies aimed at averting age-associated diseases. The clarification of innovative therapeutic targets and improvement of current interventions accompany the future of improved resilience and well-being among the older adult populace.

In general, glycation and oxidative stress have important roles as underlying mechanisms for aging processes and age-related diseases. Understanding the effects of these processes on cell physiology and organ structure to create successful approaches to preserve healthy geriatric individuals and make us immortal. With particular focus on glycation and oxidative stress, researchers seek crucial insights into novel therapeutic approaches that may have the potential to improve quality of life and reduce the plague of age-related morbidity and mortality.

6.3. Gut Microbiota Modulation: Effects on Overall Health and Longevity

The human gastrointestinal tract harbors a complex ecosystem of microorganisms collectively known as the gut microbiota. Comprising trillions of bacteria, viruses, fungi, and other microbes, the gut microbiota plays a pivotal role in maintaining various aspects of human health, including digestion, metabolism, immune function, and neurological processes. The composition and diversity of the gut microbiota are influenced by numerous factors, including diet, lifestyle, genetics, and environmental exposures.

- **Interplay Between Gut Microbiota and Health**

The dynamic relationship between the gut microbiota and human health, highlighted in the earlier discussions, enhances an equally intriguing synthesis. The act of fermentation at the gut microbiota is also invaluable in this dialogue; it is especially crucial in digesting fibers from the foods and indigestible carbohydrate. Such biochemical alchemy leads to the formation of SCFAs such as acetate, propionate, and butyrate etc. But SCFAs are so much more than just byproducts; they become key actors too they are energy for intestinal cells, masters of immunity and guardians of the shield that terrifies invading pathogens.

Significantly, the gut microbiota does not stop here; it gives immunity control the symphony of immunomodulatory griefs through tail specific species and metabolites. This regulatory function does not end with the gut, having effects on a wide array of the body's physiological aspects. The gut microbiota is delicately balanced; however, it could be a buffeted resulting in dysbiosis i.e., an imbalanced state long has been associated with many diseases. Various diseases due to gastrointestinal failure, autoimmune conditions, metabolic disorders and even the neurodegenerative conditions have been associated to disturbances in the equilibrium of the gut microbiota.

The tympanic response is augmented by the presence of increasing amounts of saturated fat and is sensitive to even small amounts of polyunsaturated fatty acids; this has been termed the 'tympanic paradox'. By harnessing this knowledge, such new and creative ways of handling and preventing a range of diseases by targeting the gut microbiota, an ally in nature bound by multiple knots with human welfare, may be created.

- **Impact of Gut Microbiota on Longevity**

This novel research trend is related to the understanding of the natural mechanisms behind the relation of the life span to gut microbiota which was discovered to possess a twofold lobated structure. A number of surveys done on different animal models have revealed striking associations between the gut microbiota and life-span. These studies highlight the central role of microbial makeup and function in controlling longevity pathways.

An important mediator accounts for how gut microbiota affects life span is by regulating inflammation and stress levels in the host animals. The dysbiosis states, in which there are imbalances in bacteria population, most often, serve as the initiators of chronic low-grade inflammation or as a symbol of inheritance and aging and its disorders. On the other hand, some of the beneficial microbes and metabolites of microbuses, possess and even exhibit powerful anti-inflammatory and anti-oxidant activity, which could slow down the aging process and support lifespan.

Additionally, the gut microbiota coordinates nutrient metabolism and energy balance, inducing tremendous impacts on host fatness, insulin responsiveness, and lipid content. However, anomalous functioning of these physiologic mechanisms can be seen as a contributing factor for the development of metabolic syndrome, obesity, type 2 diabetes, and cardiovascular diseases – important mortality risk factors.

It is important to understand the complicated functioning of gut microbiota in relation to longevity for therapeutic potential.

Treatment approaches that aim to reshape gut microbial communities via dietary changes, probiotics or fecal microbiota transplantation are novel avenues for aging beneficially and longevity promotion. With further studies in this area continuing to unravel the complex mechanisms behind the gut microbiota's contributions to longevity, the development of innovative replacement therapies that can lead to better human health and longevity is little doubt inevitable.

- **Strategies for Modulating Gut Microbiota**

Human health and life span are regulated by the complex ecosystem, gut microbiota that is the microorganisms that live in the large intestine or gastrointestinal tract. Considering its importance, there is much interest in whether influences on microbial composition and activity could bring therapeutic benefit.

The various strategies some of which include dietary interventions, prebiotics, probiotics, synbiotics, fecal microbiota transplantation (FMT) emerging with lots of promise to support healthier gut microbiota and enhance lifespan are promising.

Dietary patterns rich in fiber and fruits, vegetables, and fermented foods have shown efficacy, as they both promote the expansion of beneficial gut microbes and maintain microbiome richness. These prebiotics, specifically nondigestible fibers, would preferentially stimulate the growth and activity of probiotics, giving a nature way for the proliferation of the healthy gut microbiota. Parallel to this, probiotics, living microorganisms with established health effects, are capable of modulating microbiota' population and activity once consumed in sufficient amounts.

Thus, synbiotics is an example of a synergistic method that may be utilized to enliven the human gut micro biome communities as to also increase its medicinal potential. When various pathological conditions including severe dysbiosis or gastrointestinal diseases affect the microbiota composition and function, a powerful tool of FMT contributes to the restoration of microbial diversity and activity though transfer of healthy donor fecal microbiota to the recipient.

In conclusion, with regards to the ways of reshaping the eubiota, there are a decent number of methods that hold a potential for wellbeing and longevity. Using dietary interventions and some specific therapeutic approaches, such as prebiotics, probiotics, synbiotics, and FMT, both individuals and clinicians can play an active role in maintaining a healthy and resilient gut microbiota that facilitates longevity.

6.4. Evaluation of Acarbose as a Potential Longevity Medication

Various pharmacological interventions have also been tried in the bid to increase the longevity of humanity and foster healthy living, one of the ways is through the use of Acarbose. Acarbose is a medicine used to treat type 2 diabetes by reducing process of digestion of carbohydrates in intestinal tract. Yet, its applicability in elongating life and treating age-related diseases has drawn the interest of scientists, a considerable number of which have performed thorough studies on it.

- **Mechanism of Action:**

Acarbose's mechanism of action is rather specific and is directed to alpha-glucosidase enzymes resided within the small intestine. These enzymes are very important because they help in breakdown of the complex carbohydrates into simple sugars that can be absorbed. Acarbose contributes to the reduction of carbohydrates from a diet by inhibiting the alpha-glucosidase, which leads to a lower rate of the digestion of carbohydrates and consequent absorption. This subsequently leads to a slow release of glucose into the bloodstream and hence following meals, the surges in the blood sugar level are moderated to avoid the spikes commonly associated with meals. This machinery is highly advantageous for people with diabetes in order to reduce postprandial hyperglycemia, which is a condition that infers high blood glucose levels after meals.

The modulation of glucose metabolism by acarbose is an important mechanism of the drug's therapeutic effects. Slow absorption of carbohydrates in the body contributes to the regulation of blood sugar levels during the period of the day, which has a positive effect on glycemic control in patients with diabetes. This process not only helps to stabilize blood glucose levels but also reduces the incidence of complications associated with an uncontrolled disease, such as CVD, neuropathy and retinopathy.

-   **Impact on Glycation and Oxidative Stress:**

AGEs are post-biotic products produced following the combination of a protein or a lipid with another molecule, and this non-enzymatic reaction occurs between sugars. AGEs accumulation was described as one of the best hallmarks of aging and the initiator of various age associated diseases and complications. Tissue injury, inflammation, and oxidative stress caused by AGEs deprive the aging process of health and increase the risks of chronic disease.

The postprandial capacity of acarbose to restrict glucose peaks has a profound significance in minimizing AGE buildup. Acarbose thereby limits the rapid and large influx of glucose into the bloodstream after meals and consequently helps reduce the susceptible substrate that is available in glycation reactions. As a result, the AGEs formation and accumulation processes gets slowed down, thus helping in reducing the glycation-specific tissue and organ damage laden burden.

In addition, through its effects on glucose metabolism, Acarbose may serve to reduce indirectly oxidative stress, a process that is ultimately marked by a mismatch between the formation of reactive oxygen species and a body's available antioxidant defenses. Hence, once Acarbose standardizes blood glucose levels and suppresses fluctuations, it minimizes the oxidative stress connected with hyperglycemia, and through such protective mechanisms, this drug influences age-related degenerative processes.

- **Influence on Gut Microbiota**

Gut microbiota is a large and diverse microbial population occupying the GI tract and has profound influences on the human health and metabolism. Among the identified mechanisms believed to influence gut microbiota, Acarbose, an antihyperglycemic agent and commonly used treatment for management of hyperglycemia in patients with diabetes, is associated to modulate microbial composition and function.

Acarbose acts by inhibiting the absorption of carbohydrates into the intestine, lowering the sugars from the diet available to the bacteria for fermentation and absorption. This modified substrate availability leads to a less favorable environment for the propagation of sugar-dependent pathogenic organisms but favors beneficial bacteria that can convert more complicated substrates such as fiber into useful forms. As a result, Acarbose causes a preferred composition of the gut microbiota with improved microbial diversity and higher abundance of health-beneficial taxa.

Besides, Acarbose-linked shifts in gut microbiota involve more than a mere altering of their composition. The impacts of the drug on carbohydrate metabolism and pathways of fermentation lead metabolic adaptations within the microbial community, which are involved in improving metabolic homeostasis and decreasing inflammation. In turn, these microbial changes can result in alterations to the physiology of the host, potentially decreasing the risk for metabolic disorders, supporting a general state of good health and increased longevity.

All in all, the research results suggest that Acarbose is a promising approach to modulate the composition as well as the function of gut microbiome that impacts metabolic health and longevity outcomes.

- ## **Clinical Evidence and Observations:**

Animal and clinical evidence has jointly provided a positive picture regarding the potential longevity of Acarbose. It was demonstrated through animal studies on different model organisms such as nematodes, fruit flies, and rodents that the addition of supplement Acarbose increases the period of life and can improve healthy aging. These variables were associated with Acarbose acting as a dietary restriction mimetic which is a well-known intervention with increased life spans across species. In preclinical models Acarbose protects from advanced age and pathogenesis by modulating crucial metabolic pathways involved in aging and longevity.

In clinical trials, efficacy of Acarbose has been shown for the beneficial effects on glycemic control and cardiovascular risk factors in impaired glucose tolerant subjects or those with type 2 diabetes. Although there are not many longitudinal studies evaluating the effects of Acarbose on lifespan and age-related morbidity, the advantages of this drug impact on metabolic parameters, vascular health have shown the possible use of Acarbose in healthy aging.

Overall, though additional studies are necessary to detail the long-term effects of Acarbose on lifespan and aging trajectories, current data confirms its efficacy in achieving ameliorated metabolic homeostasis and improving human longevity.

- **<u>Considerations and Future Directions</u>**

As promising as it is on the road to being a longevity drug, Acarbose is not above its limitations and concerns. The major and frequently reported side effects of Acarbose use are adverse gastrointestinal side effects and these include flatulence, bloating, and diarrhea and these side effects may limit tolerability in some patients. In addition, more clinical trials and epidemiologic studies are required to understand the lasting outcomes of Acarbose on old age or outcomes relating to mortality.

However, further studies should focus on better understanding the mechanisms of action by which Acarbose promotes longevity and the definition of the best dosing schedule and patient population receiving its treatment. Moreover, the examination of possible synergies with Acarbose and other interventions: dietary modifications, exercise, and other pharmacological agents may increase efficacy in improving healthy aging and increasing life expectancy.

Summing up, Acarbose can act as a probable long-life agent due to its impact of glucose metabolism regulation, oxidative stress reduction, and modulation of the gut microbiome. While additional studies are needed to fully characterize its lifespan-prolonging properties and counter the highlighted limitations, Acarbose shows significant potential in promoting health aging and longevity.

CHAPTER 7
ASSESSING LONGEVITY MEDICATIONS

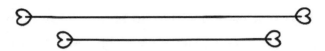

7.1. Comparative Analysis of Rapamycin, Metformin, and Acarbose

Throughout the attempt to obtain better longevity and vitality, pharmacology has found its way of minimizing the effects of aging with a goal of promoting general health. Some of the compounds that have come under intense consideration include Rapamycin, Metformin, and Acarbose. All these drugs act through different pathways and separately provide for different prospects, advantages and concerns in developing more life span and health span.

We are studying molecular pathways, clinical uses as well as the advantages and disadvantages of Rapamycin, Metformin, and Acarbose in longevity science.

- ## **Rapamycin: Targeting the mTOR Pathway**

Rapamycin, which was initially acquired as an immunosuppressant, has come out as an emerging drug for promoting longevity through its intervention in the mTOR pathway. The mTOR pathway represents a crucial regulator of cellular growth, metabolism and aging processes, wherein it is activated by available nutrients, growth factors, and cellular energy levels. As such through inhibiting the mTOR, Rapamycin imitates nutritional restriction regulation that triggers a chain of biological reactions that are associated with longevity and good quality of living.

An important mechanism responding to Rapamycin longevity effects is the decreasing in proteins synthesis and the promotion of autophagy – a process of cellular clearing up of damaged parts and renewing cells. Furthermore, Rapamycin can increase metabolic regulation, making it possible to postpone age-related diseases as cardiovascular or neurodegenerative conditions, or types of cancer.

Although Rapamycin can be a valuable treatment, it is associated with challenges in terms of its side effect profile as well as long-term safety aspects. In the case of long-term use of Rapamycin, significant adverse effects such as immunosuppression, metabolic dysregulation and increased infections have been observed thus, in the clinical setting, it always warrants close monitoring and risk-benefit assessment.

- ## Metformin: Targeting Metabolic Pathways

Metformin, a widely used medication for managing type 2 diabetes, has garnered attention for its potential longevity benefits beyond glycemic control. The primary mechanism of action of Metformin involves the activation of AMP-activated protein kinase (AMPK), a key regulator of cellular energy metabolism. AMPK activation improves cellular energy efficiency and mimics the effects of caloric restriction, promoting longevity through enhanced metabolic regulation and reduced oxidative stress.

In addition to its effects on metabolic pathways, Metformin has been shown to mitigate chronic inflammation, a hallmark of aging, by modulating inflammatory signaling pathways and reducing the production of pro-inflammatory cytokines. These anti-inflammatory properties contribute to Metformin's potential in preventing age-related diseases and promoting overall health span.

Despite its well-established safety profile and widespread use in clinical practice, Metformin may be associated with gastrointestinal side effects such as nausea, diarrhea, and abdominal discomfort in some individuals. Furthermore, ongoing research is needed to elucidate the long-term effects of Metformin on aging and to identify optimal dosing regimens for longevity promotion.

- **Acarbose: Modulating Glucose Metabolism and Beyond**

Carbohydrate breakdown is decreased by acarbose that is widely used in the management of type 2 diabetes, and thus, there is slower absorption of carbohydrates in the intestinal lumen, which reduces the peaks of glycemia that occur after the meal. It has been shown to be involved in the regulation of glucose metabolism, lowering glycosylation and oxidative stress, and positively impacting gut microbiota composition, in addition to its glucose control properties.

The antiaging potential of Acarbose may be attributed to two fundamental effects: it minimizes the negative impact of hyperglycemia on cellular function and slows down the aging process through functional pathways. Acarbose lowers glycation and oxidative stress and may thus prevent age-specific complications such as cardiovascular disorders, dementia, and retinopathy.

Possible benefits of a treatment with Acarbose include side effects most likely to be experienced by the gastrointestinal tract such as flatulence, bloating, and diarrhea that may reduce its tolerability and adherence in some patients. Moreover, additional studies are required to clarify the wide range spectrum of Acarbose actions on the aging process and for better development its practical use in prolonging the aging process and health span.

To wrap up, Rapamycin, Metformin, and Acarbose can be seen as promising directions of achieving longevity and vitality by using pharmacological means. Although every drug target specific molecular pathways and works by a different mechanism of action, all of them aim to regulate age-related processes along with associated diseases. As sustainability in the field of longevity science continues to progress, clarification of the advantages and constraints of these medications will be critical to the utilization of their full potential to enhance the aging process and lead to a longer lifespan.

7.2. Potential Benefits and Limitations of Pharmacological Approaches to Longevity

Life extension efforts, the discovery of allostatic mechanisms, and challenges to healthspan-aging though inspired pharmacological strategies, as it is one of the most promising ways for research and intervention. Development of these strategies includes the use and manipulation of medications that impact underlying biological processes such as aging and age-related ailments. Although these pharmacological interventions provide a complementary approach to improving the life expectancy of human beings, some critical limitations and challenges for their adoption in practice emerge.

- Potential Benefits

1. Targeted Intervention in Aging Processes

Pharmacological approaches to longevity target specific biological pathways implicated in aging and age-related diseases. For example, medications such as Rapamycin, Metformin, and Acarbose act on molecular pathways involved in cellular metabolism, inflammation, and oxidative stress.

By modulating these pathways, these medications have the potential to delay the onset of age-related decline and improve overall health outcomes.

2. Delaying Age-Related Diseases

One of the primary objectives of pharmacological interventions in longevity is to delay the onset and progression of age-related diseases such as cardiovascular disease, diabetes, and neurodegenerative disorders. By targeting underlying mechanisms of aging, these medications may help mitigate the risk factors associated with these diseases, thereby promoting healthier aging and extending lifespan.

3. Improving Quality of Life

In addition to extending lifespan, pharmacological approaches to longevity aim to improve the quality of life in aging populations. By addressing age-related physiological changes and functional decline, these medications have the potential to enhance physical and cognitive function, preserve independence, and promote overall well-being in older adults.

4. Complementary to Lifestyle Interventions

Pharmacological interventions in longevity are often viewed as complementary to lifestyle interventions such as healthy diet, regular exercise, and stress management. While lifestyle factors play a crucial role in promoting longevity, pharmacological approaches offer additional support in addressing underlying biological processes associated with aging, thereby synergistically enhancing the effects of healthy lifestyle practices.

-   **Potential Limitations**

1. Side Effects and Safety Concerns

One of the primary limitations of pharmacological interventions in longevity is the potential for adverse side effects and safety concerns associated with long-term medication use. Many longevity medications, including Rapamycin and Metformin, may cause gastrointestinal disturbances, metabolic alterations, or other undesirable effects, which may outweigh their potential benefits in certain individuals.

2. Lack of Long-Term Data

Another challenge in evaluating the efficacy and safety of pharmacological approaches to longevity is the limited availability of long-term clinical data. While some medications have demonstrated promising results in preclinical studies and short-term clinical trials, their effects over extended periods of time and in diverse populations remain largely unknown.

Longitudinal studies are needed to assess the sustained efficacy and safety profile of these medications in real-world settings.

3. *Individual Variability in Response*

Individual variability in response to pharmacological interventions presents another limitation in the field of longevity research. Factors such as genetic predisposition, underlying health conditions, and lifestyle factors can influence an individual's response to medication, making it challenging to predict and optimize treatment outcomes for all patients.

4. *Ethical and Societal Considerations*

The use of pharmacological interventions in longevity raises ethical and societal considerations regarding equity, access, and resource allocation. There are concerns about the equitable distribution of longevity medications, especially in disadvantaged populations, as well as the potential for widening health disparities based on socioeconomic factors.

Pharmacological approaches to longevity hold significant promise in extending lifespan, delaying age-related diseases, and improving quality of life in aging populations. However, they also pose inherent limitations and challenges that must be carefully addressed through rigorous research, clinical monitoring, and ethical deliberation. By advancing our understanding of the potential benefits and limitations of pharmacological interventions, we can strive towards a more holistic and personalized approach to promoting healthy aging and longevity in diverse populations.

7.3. Ethical Considerations and Societal Implications of Extending Lifespan

Extending human lifespan is a compelling prospect that has captured the imagination of scientists, ethicists, policymakers, and the general public alike. As advancements in medical science and technology continue to push the boundaries of what is possible, questions surrounding the ethical implications and broader societal impacts of extending lifespan become increasingly pertinent.

- **Ethical Dilemmas in Lifespan Extension**

The pursuit of extending human lifespan raises a host of ethical dilemmas that warrant careful consideration. At the forefront is the question of equity and access. If lifespan extension therapies become available, who will have access to them? Will they be affordable and accessible to all individuals, regardless of socioeconomic status, or will they exacerbate existing disparities in healthcare access?

Another ethical concern is the potential for exacerbating overpopulation and resource scarcity. Extending lifespan without addressing underlying issues of resource distribution and environmental sustainability could strain finite resources and exacerbate social and environmental challenges.

- **<u>Quality vs. Quantity of Life</u>**

Beyond the ethical considerations surrounding access and resource allocation, there is a fundamental question about the quality versus quantity of life. While extending lifespan holds the promise of prolonged existence, it does not necessarily guarantee a higher quality of life. Ethical frameworks must prioritize not just extending lifespan but also enhancing the healthspan—the period of life free from disease and disability.

- **<u>Implications for Healthcare Systems</u>**

Extending lifespan also has significant implications for healthcare systems worldwide. As populations age and life expectancy increases, healthcare systems must adapt to meet the evolving needs of aging populations. This includes addressing chronic diseases, age-related conditions, and providing comprehensive care for older adults.

Furthermore, the increasing demand for healthcare services may strain existing infrastructure and resources, necessitating innovative solutions to improve efficiency, accessibility, and affordability of healthcare delivery.

- **Social and Cultural Shifts**

Extending lifespan can precipitate profound social and cultural shifts. Traditional notions of aging, retirement, and intergenerational relationships may undergo transformation as individuals live longer, healthier lives. The concept of a "career" may evolve, with individuals pursuing multiple careers over an extended lifespan.

Moreover, extended lifespans may challenge existing social structures and norms, including family dynamics, marriage patterns, and intergenerational wealth transfer. Intergenerational equity and the balance of power between generations may become increasingly salient issues in society.

- **Moral and Philosophical Reflections**

Ethical considerations surrounding lifespan extension invite profound moral and philosophical reflections. Questions about the meaning and purpose of life, the nature of suffering and death, and the value of human existence become central to discussions about extending lifespan.

From a philosophical standpoint, proponents of lifespan extension argue for the inherent value of life and the moral imperative to alleviate suffering and promote well-being. Critics, however, caution against the potential hubris of humans seeking to transcend the natural limits of existence and warn against unintended consequences that may accompany efforts to extend lifespan.

The effort to prolong the lives of humans indeed offers the much-sophisticated weave of issues to be ethically considered and the effects that may result in the somewhere culture. In direct response to the continued redefinition of the limits of man's life by technological advancements, the world must focus on serious introspection regarding the moral assessment of lifespan extension.

Longer life requires careful balance of equitable, high-quality life, and societal coherence to ensure active involvement of all stakeholders and the society as a whole. In the end, it is the ethical commitment to good life and human beings' quality of life that deserve principally human rights and equity that should drive our collective attempts to lengthen lifespan to be appropriate, unbiased and steady.

**7.4.   Future   Directions   in   Longevity   Research:
Exploring the Quest for Enhanced Vitality**

In the world of longevity research, longevity prevails as an ideal
for scientific conduct inciting inquiries into prolonged life and
better health. It seems that our knowledge about the aging
mechanisms continues to deepen and the technological progress
keeps to accelerate, while more and more researchers set out to
explore what has long been considered someone else's territory
and yet it is possible to find new paths of longevity or even to
contemplate the reversal of the aging processes.

-   <u>**Understanding the Aging Process**</u>

At the core of longevity research lies the quest to unravel the
mysteries of aging. Scientists delve into the intricate biochemical
pathways and genetic determinants that underpin the aging
process, seeking insights into how and why our bodies age.

By deciphering the molecular mechanisms driving aging,
researchers aim to develop interventions capable of slowing,
halting, or even reversing age-related degeneration.

- **<u>Targeting Cellular Senescence</u>**

One emerging frontier in longevity research focuses on cellular senescence – the phenomenon where cells cease to divide and enter a state of irreversible growth arrest. Senescent cells accumulate with age and contribute to tissue dysfunction and chronic inflammation, hallmarks of aging and age-related diseases. Scientists are exploring novel strategies to selectively eliminate senescent cells, known as senolytics, with the goal of rejuvenating tissues and extending healthy lifespan.

- **<u>Harnessing the Power of Regenerative Medicine</u>**

Regenerative medicine holds immense promise in the quest for enhanced vitality. Researchers investigate the potential of stem cells, tissue engineering, and regenerative therapies to repair and regenerate damaged organs and tissues. By harnessing the body's innate regenerative capacity, scientists envision a future where age-related degeneration can be reversed, restoring function and vitality to aging tissues and organs.

- **<u>Unraveling the Secrets of Genetics and Epigenetics</u>**

Advancements in genomic and epigenomic research provide valuable insights into the genetic and epigenetic determinants of aging. Scientists study the genetic variations and epigenetic modifications associated with longevity and age-related diseases, identifying key genetic pathways and molecular markers that influence aging trajectories. By unraveling the secrets encoded within our DNA and epigenome, researchers aim to develop precision therapies tailored to individual genetic profiles, optimizing healthspan and lifespan.

- **Exploring the Role of Metabolic Health**

Metabolic health emerges as a critical determinant of longevity, with metabolic dysregulation linked to an increased risk of age-related diseases such as diabetes, cardiovascular disease, and neurodegeneration. Researchers investigate the intricate interplay between metabolism, aging, and longevity, exploring metabolic pathways, dietary interventions, and pharmacological strategies to promote metabolic health and delay the onset of age-related decline.

- **Leveraging Artificial Intelligence and Big Data**

In the era of big data and artificial intelligence (AI), researchers harness the power of computational tools and machine learning algorithms to analyze vast datasets and uncover hidden patterns in aging and longevity. AI-driven approaches enable researchers to identify novel drug targets, predict therapeutic outcomes, and personalize interventions based on individual health profiles, accelerating the pace of discovery and innovation in longevity research.

- **Integrating Lifestyle Interventions with Longevity Strategies**

While scientific breakthroughs pave the way for enhanced longevity, the importance of lifestyle interventions cannot be overstated. Researchers emphasize the role of healthy lifestyle practices – including balanced nutrition, regular exercise, stress management, and adequate sleep – in promoting longevity and vitality. Integrating lifestyle interventions with cutting-edge longevity strategies offers a holistic approach to aging well, empowering individuals to proactively enhance their healthspan and quality of life.

The future of longevity research holds boundless potential, fueled by interdisciplinary collaboration, technological innovation, and a deepening understanding of the aging process. As scientists venture into uncharted territories and explore novel frontiers, the quest for enhanced vitality continues to inspire hope and promise for a healthier, more vibrant future.

CONCLUSION

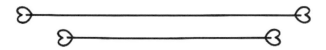

In the pages of "Longevity: In "Future of Enhanced Lifespans and Vitality," we set out on a path through the complex interplay of aging, health, and emerging breakthroughs transforming longevity science. Having reached the end of this discussion, it is pertinent to reflect on the principal insights that have been garnered and encourage readers to take proactive steps in improving their health and lifespan.

- **<u>Recap of Key Insights:</u>**

Throughout our discourse, we delved into the multifaceted dynamics underlying the aging process and the pivotal role lifestyle practices play in shaping our health trajectories. From the foundational pillars of diet, exercise, stress management, and sleep hygiene to the intricate mechanisms governing longevity medications, our understanding of the determinants of health and vitality has expanded exponentially.

In dissecting the mechanisms of longevity medications such as Rapamycin, Metformin, and Acarbose, we unraveled the intricate molecular pathways that hold promise in extending lifespan and ameliorating age-related ailments. From Rapamycin's modulation of the mTOR pathway to Metformin's activation of AMPK and Acarbose's influence on glucose metabolism, each medication offers a glimpse into the pharmacological interventions reshaping the aging paradigm. Moreover, we grappled with the nuances of ethical considerations and the need for a balanced approach in navigating the intersection of science, medicine, and human longevity. As we stand on the precipice of unprecedented breakthroughs, it is imperative to exercise prudence and circumspection in harnessing the transformative potential of longevity science for the betterment of humanity.

- **<u>Encouragement for Readers:</u>**

Armed with newfound knowledge and insights, readers are implored to embark on a journey of self-discovery and empowerment in prioritizing their health and longevity. The revelations gleaned from "Longevity" serve as a clarion call to action, inspiring individuals to embrace proactive measures and forge a path towards optimal well-being.

First and foremost, it is essential to cultivate a mindset of mindfulness and intentionality in our daily choices and habits. By embracing the tenets of healthy living—nourishing our bodies with nutrient-dense foods, engaging in regular physical activity, managing stress effectively, and prioritizing restorative sleep—we lay the foundation for a resilient and vibrant existence.

Furthermore, the insights garnered from our exploration of longevity medications underscore the transformative potential of pharmacological interventions in augmenting human healthspan. While the allure of extending lifespan is undeniable, it is imperative to approach such interventions with caution and discernment, mindful of the potential risks and uncertainties inherent in medical innovation. In the pursuit of longevity, it is equally imperative to foster a holistic approach that encompasses not only physical health but also mental, emotional, and spiritual well-being. Cultivating meaningful connections, nurturing a sense of purpose, and engaging in practices that nourish the soul are integral facets of the longevity journey.

In closing, "Longevity" serves as a beacon of hope and possibility, illuminating the path towards a future where individuals can thrive and flourish well into their golden years. As we bid adieu to these pages, let us embark on this journey with courage, curiosity, and unwavering resolve, knowing that the pursuit of health and longevity is not merely a destination but a lifelong odyssey of self-discovery and transformation.

May we embrace the boundless potential that resides within us, and may our collective efforts pave the way for a world where health, vitality, and longevity are accessible to all.

With gratitude and optimism,

Viktor

Made in United States
Troutdale, OR
04/08/2024